NURSING PHOTOBOOK™
Giving Cardiac Care

NURSING83 BOOKS™
SPRINGHOUSE CORPORATION
SPRINGHOUSE, PENNSYLVANIA

NURSING83 BOOKS™

NURSING PHOTOBOOK™ SERIES
Providing Respiratory Care
Managing I.V. Therapy
Dealing with Emergencies
Giving Medications
Assessing Your Patients
Using Monitors
Providing Early Mobility
Giving Cardiac Care
Performing GI Procedures
Implementing Urologic Procedures
Controlling Infection
Ensuring Intensive Care
Coping with Neurologic Disorders
Caring for Surgical Patients
Working with Orthopedic Patients
Nursing Pediatric Patients
Helping Geriatric Patients
Attending Ob/Gyn Patients
Aiding Ambulatory Patients
Carrying Out Special Procedures

NURSING SKILLBOOK® SERIES
Dealing with Death and Dying
Reading EKGs Correctly
Managing Diabetics Properly
Assessing Vital Functions Accurately
Helping Cancer Patients Effectively
Giving Cardiovascular Drugs Safely
Giving Emergency Care Competently
Monitoring Fluid and Electrolytes Precisely
Documenting Patient Care Responsibly
Combatting Cardiovascular Diseases Skillfully
Coping with Neurologic Problems Proficiently
Nursing Critically Ill Patients Confidently
Using Crisis Intervention Wisely

NURSE'S REFERENCE LIBRARY®
Diseases
Diagnostics
Drugs
Assessment
Procedures
Definitions

Nursing83 DRUG HANDBOOK™

NURSING PHOTOBOOK™ Series
PUBLISHER
Eugene W. Jackson

EDITORIAL DIRECTOR
Jean Robinson

CLINICAL DIRECTOR
Barbara McVan, RN

ART DIRECTOR
Lisa A. Gilde

**Springhouse Corporation
Book Division**
DIRECTOR
Timothy B. King

DIRECTOR, RESEARCH
Elizabeth O'Brien

VICE-PRESIDENT, PRODUCTION AND PURCHASING
Bacil Guiley

Staff for this volume
BOOK EDITOR
Richard Samuel West

CLINICAL EDITOR
Helene Ritting Nawrocki, RN

ASSOCIATE EDITOR
Katherine W. Carey

PHOTOGRAPHER
Paul A. Cohen

ASSOCIATE DESIGNERS
Linda Jovinelly Franklin
Carol Stickles

ASSISTANT PHOTOGRAPHER
Thomas Staudenmayer

EDITORIAL/GRAPHIC COORDINATOR
Doreen K. Stowers

CLINICAL/GRAPHIC COORDINATOR
Evelyn M. James

COPY EDITOR
Eric R. Rinehimer

EDITORIAL STAFF ASSISTANT
Cynthia A. O'Connell

PHOTOGRAPHY ASSISTANT
Frank Margeson

ART PRODUCTION MANAGER
Wilbur D. Davidson

ARTISTS
Darcy Feralio   Louise Stamper
Diane Fox   Joan Walsh
Robert Perry   Ron Yablon
Sandra Simms

TYPOGRAPHY MANAGER
David C. Kosten

ASSISTANT TO THE
TYPOGRAPHY MANAGER
David W. Davenport

TYPOGRAPHY ASSISTANTS
Ethel Halle
Diane Paluba

PRODUCTION MANAGERS
Robert L. Dean, Jr.
Kathy Murphy

ASSISTANT PRODUCTION MANAGER
Deborah C. Meiris

PRODUCTION ASSISTANT
Donald G. Knauss

ILLUSTRATORS
Bill Edwards   Robert Jackson
Jack Freas   Henry Rothman
Jean Gardner   Nancy Schill
Bob Hambly   Bud Yingling
Tom Herbert

SERIES GRAPHIC DESIGNER
John C. Isely

COVER PHOTO
Seymour Mednick

**Clinical consultants
for this volume**

Alyce Lanoue, RN, BSN, MSN, CCRN
Cardiovascular Clinical Specialist
Norwood Hospital
Norwood, Mass.

Connie Slay, RN, BSN, MSN
Cardiovascular Clinical Specialist
Crozer-Chester Medical Center
Chester, Pa.

Amended reprint, 1983
© 1983, 1981 by Springhouse Corporation,
1111 Bethlehem Pike, Springhouse, Pa. 19477
All rights reserved. Reproduction in whole or part by any means whatsoever without written permission of the publisher is prohibited by law.
Printed in the United States of America.
PB-051083

Library of Congress Cataloging in Publication Data

Main entry under title:

Giving cardiac care.

(Nursing Photobook Series)
"Nursing81 books."
Bibliography: p.
Includes index.
1. Heart—Diseases—Nursing. I. Springhouse Corporation
[DNLM: 1. Cardiology—Nursing texts. 2. Heart diseases—Nursing. WY 152.5 G539]
RC674.G58   610.73'69   80-27519
ISBN 0-916730-28-X

Contents

Contributors

At the time of original publication, these contributors held the following positions.

Elizabeth Billet is a pediatric clinical nurse specialist at UCLA Medical Center in Los Angeles. She received her BSN from Marquette University, Milwaukee, and her MA from UCLA.

Sheila Cross is a nursing coordinator and medical/surgical nursing teacher at Vanier College, Montreal. After earning her nursing diploma from Foothills Hospital, Calgary, Alberta, she received her BN from McGill University in Montreal. She is currently enrolled at McGill University in the Faculty of Education, pursuing a diploma in college teaching.

Beverly H. Cridland is associate director of nurses at Little Company of Mary Hospital in Torrance, Calif. She received her nursing diploma from St. Luke's School of Nursing, San Francisco, and her BA from Pepperdine University in Los Angeles.

Jeanne Fitzpatrick is a clinical specialist in pediatric cardiology at UCLA Medical Center in Los Angeles. Currently an MSN candidate at UCLA, she received her BSN from Mount St. Mary's College in Los Angeles. She is also a CCRN.

Barbara A. Gleeson is a cardiac rehabilitation nurse specialist at Albert Einstein Medical Center, Daroff Division, in Philadelphia. She received her BSN and MSN degrees from the University of Pennsylvania, also in Philadelphia. Previously, she had earned her nursing diploma from the Hospital of the University of Pennsylvania. She is president of the Southeastern Pennsylvania Chapter of the American Association of Critical-Care Nurses.

Alyce Souden Lanoue, an adviser for this PHOTOBOOK, is a cardiovascular clinical specialist at Norwood (Mass.) Hospital. After earning her nursing diploma at Beth Israel Hospital in Boston, she received her BSN from Boston College and her MSN from Boston University. She is also a CCRN.

Albert F. Mutton, Jr. is an instructor of respiratory therapy technology at Forsyth Technical Institute in Winston-Salem, N.C. He received his BS and MS degrees from East Tennessee State University in Johnson City. A member of the National Society of Cardiopulmonary Technology, he's a registered cardiopulmonary technologist.

Claudia Pohling is marketing services coordinator for Coratomic, Inc. in Indiana, Pa. She is an RN, who received her ASN from Rochester (Minn.) Community College.

Connie Slay, also an adviser for this PHOTOBOOK, is a clinical specialist in cardiovascular nursing at Crozer-Chester Medical Center, Chester, Pa. She received her nursing diploma from Indiana (Pa.) Hospital. She earned her BSN from Case Western Reserve in Cleveland and her MSN from the University of Pennsylvania in Philadelphia.

Arlene B. Strong is a cardiac clinical specialist at the Veterans Administration Medical Center in Portland, Ore. She received a BSN from the University of Portland, and an MN from the University of Oregon. She's also an adult nurse practitioner.

Nancy Wiedemer is a cardiac rehabilitation specialist at Albert Einstein Medical Center, Daroff Division, in Philadelphia. She earned her diploma from Fitzgerald Mercy Hospital School of Nursing, in Darby, Pa. After graduating from Boston College with a BSN, she received her MSN from the University of Pennsylvania in Philadelphia.

Introduction

Caring for a cardiac patient goes beyond any one speciality. If you want to give expert cardiac care, you must know about a wide variety of procedures, such as radiography, hardwire monitoring, defibrillation, and exercise EKGs. How can you hope to understand all you need to know? It's not easy. A good education and practice are the best ways. Reading on your own will help, too.

That's where this PHOTOBOOK comes in. We've designed it to act as your guide through the maze of cardiac care procedures. We begin where you'd begin—interviewing the patient to compile his medical history. This may sound unexciting. But it's important, because you can't leave any stones unturned in your effort to gather patient information. If you follow the instructions contained in the dozens of pages we devote to this subject, you'll develop an information file so useful that you'll rely on it daily.

The myriad of diagnostic tests that the doctor may order can be very confusing. That's why we've divided them into five distinct groupings. In our cardiography pages, you'll find out what 12-lead electrocardiography and vectorcardiography have in common and how they differ. Then, you'll learn about radiography—what it is and how it works. After that, we'll explore sonic testing and tell you what you need to know about phonocardiography and echocardiography. Taking a pulse wave tracing and an apexcardiogram are covered too. Finally, you'll learn the how's and why's of cardiac catheterization.

The doctor will probably order continuous cardiac monitoring. For the patient on bed rest, that means hardwire system. If your patient's ambulatory, you'll connect him to a telemetry monitor.

As you know, cardiac care may not go smoothly. That's why we review emergency techniques such as cardiopulmonary resuscitation (CPR), countershock therapy, rotating tourniquets, and intra-aortic balloon insertion. You'll also find a dozen pages devoted to the pacemaker—how it works, and how you can make it work for your patient.

The final important phase in cardiac care is helping your patient back to good health. You'll learn about a variety of rehabilitation techniques and probably find some that are right for your patient.

As we've said, providing competent cardiac care isn't simple. But, we believe, if you read this PHOTOBOOK carefully and refer to it frequently, you'll find the task's easier than you thought.

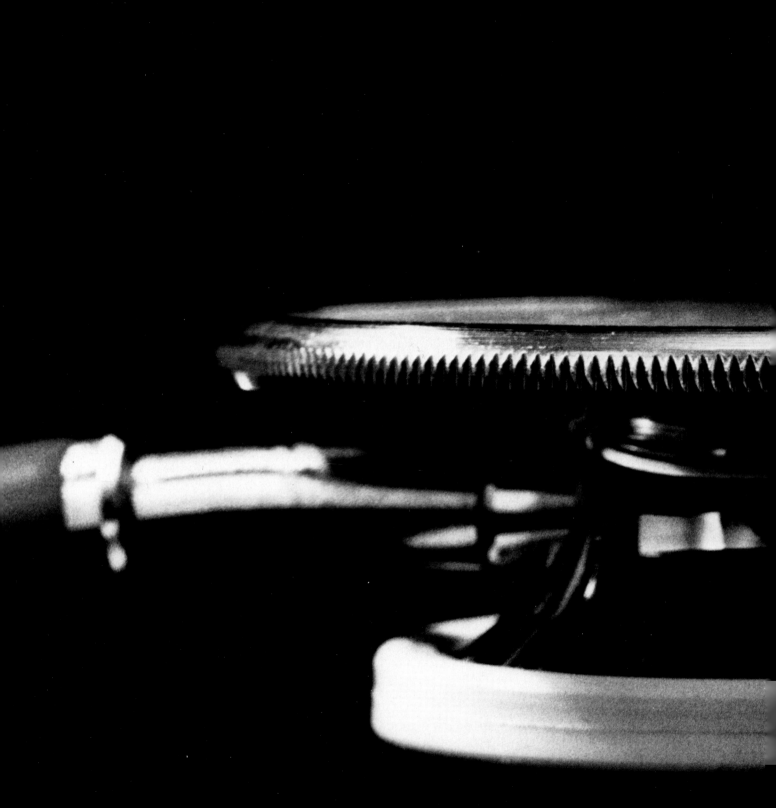

Examining Your Patient

Cardiac assessment

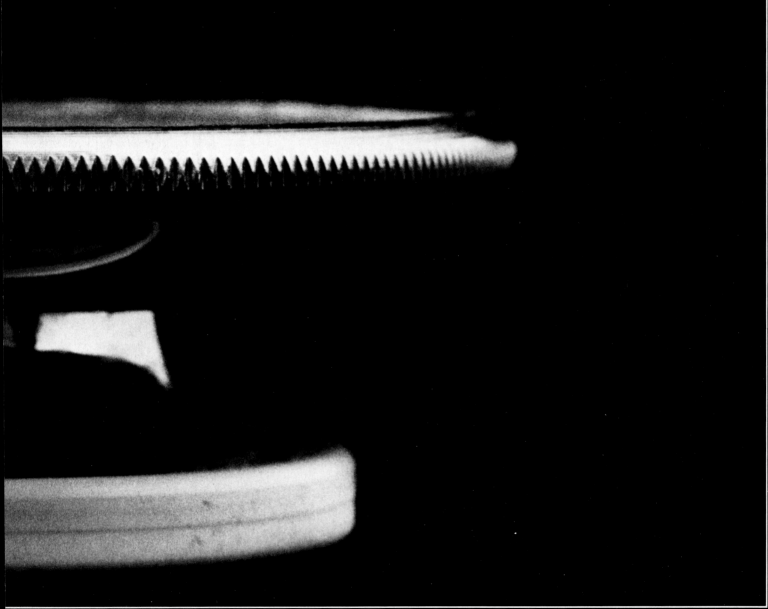

Cardiac assessment

A cardiac assessment is more than a collection of facts. It's a vital tool that you and other health-care professionals can use to give your patient the best care possible. A complete cardiac assessment breaks down into these basic steps:

• First, you'll compile your patient's medical history, focusing on his current complaint and what may have caused it.

• Then, you'll assess his circulatory system, checking his arterial pulses and his arterial and venous blood pressures.

• Next comes an inspection of his thorax and lungs, with emphasis on identifying normal and abnormal breath sounds.

• Finally, you'll conduct a thorough examination of the heart. You'll start by inspecting, palpating, and percussing to assess blood flow, and to determine heart location and size. Then, you'll auscultate to record heart sounds.

This multiphase examination reveals—in detail—the condition of your patient's cardiovascular system. However, it's too time consuming to complete if your patient's in severe pain. In such a case, simply take his vital signs and perform an electrocardiogram (EKG). Then, the doctor can diagnose your patient's cardiac problem swiftly and prescribe treatment. Later, when your patient is resting more comfortably, you can begin the detailed cardiac assessment.

For a step-by-step explanation of what a complete cardiac assessment involves, plus instructions on assessing the pediatric patient, read the following pages.

Taking your patient's medical history

History-taking may seem like a perfunctory task. But, it's an essential part of assessment that demands detectivelike skills of observation and questioning. Part of your assessment involves factual information. If your patient's unconscious or can't talk for some reason, find out this information from a friend or member of his family. But, remember to document the name of the person giving the information on the patient's record.

The other part of your assessment involves picking up subtle clues about the patient's self-image, expectations, beliefs, and family life. This between-the-lines information will help you design a care plan to fit his unique needs. Here's how to begin:

Assessment information	Your written notes (sample)	Your mental notes (sample)
Identify the patient. Write down his name, age, sex, race, nationality, marital status, occupation, and source of referral.	Louis Pantelli is a 46-year-old white male. He's an American citizen of Italian ancestry. He's married, has two sons, and works as a neighborhood grocery store manager. He was referred to the hospital by Dr. Michael Trent.	Note Mr. Pantelli's occupation. Small businesses may not provide adequate hospitalization or disability benefits. You may have to refer him to the social services department for financial assistance.
Identify the problem. Ask the patient to identify his chief complaint. Then, find out if he's experiencing any other discomfort. Include all details of his complaint, and be specific. Begin at the onset of discomfort. Ask him when the discomfort began, and what he was doing at the time. If he's taking any medication (including any over-the-counter drug) find out what it is.	Mr. Pantelli complains of a "heavy, squeezing kind of pain" in the left side of his chest, which radiates to his left jaw and down his left arm. This pain is accompanied by labored breathing, sweating, and anxiety. The pain began suddenly at 11:00 this morning, while Mr. Pantelli was lifting cartons at work. Immediately thereafter, he lay down in his office while one of his employees called Mrs. Pantelli and Dr. Trent. Dr. Trent advised that Mr. Pantelli be brought to the E.D. immediately. Mrs. Pantelli says her husband is usually stoic about pain, and rarely admits that he	Consider Mrs. Pantelli's remarks. Because of Mr. Pantelli's stoic nature, you can't assume he'll admit to discomfort or pain. This may also prove an important factor during cardiac rehabilitation.

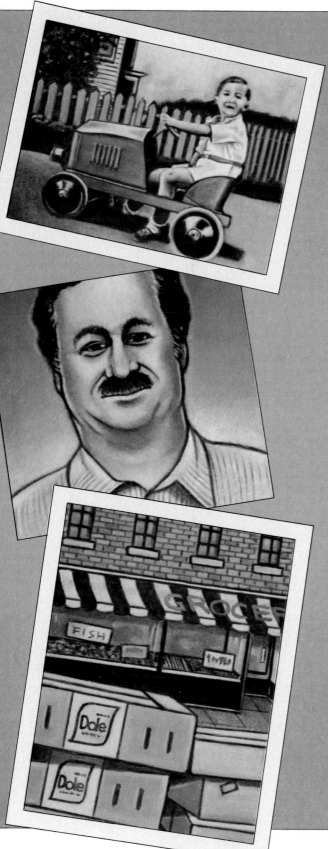

Assessment information	Your written notes (sample)	Your mental notes (sample)
	needs help. Mr. Pantelli has been given 5 mg morphine I.V. and is resting comfortably.	
Record patient history. You should record all of the patient's previous illnesses, injuries, and other medical conditions, with diagnoses, dates, and complications. You should also record allergies, current medications, and immunizations, if pertinent. If your patient's a woman, ask if she has taken or is taking birth-control pills. They may contribute to coronary artery disease (CAD).	Patient's previous illnesses: 1972 - Appendectomy with peritonitis; 1976 - Hypertension, currently being treated with 40 mg propranolol (Inderal) q.i.d. He denies any previous episodes of chest pain. He is about 20 pounds overweight. He smoked approximately 2 packs of cigarettes a day until he quit completely 3 years ago. He is allergic to penicillin.	As a former smoker, Mr. Pantelli probably has some lung damage. Keep an eye on his breath sounds and on how much oxygen he receives. Also, consider that Mr. Pantelli developed a cardiac problem even though he was receiving 40 mg Inderal q.i.d. Suspect coronary artery disease.
Record family history. Find out about the patient's familial medical history so you can assess possible precipitating hereditary factors. At that time, you may also learn if the patient is suffering any stress induced by family situations. Include the current age and state of health of patient's immediate family members. Also, record the cause of death of any immediate family member. Ask about familial diseases that may affect your patient's cardiovascular system, such as diabetes, heart disease, and blood coagulation disorders.	Mr. Pantelli's father died of congestive heart failure at age 58. His mother, age 78, has lived with Mr. Pantelli and his family for 7 years. His wife, age 43, is in good health, although she smokes a pack of cigarettes a day. His sons, ages 18 and 16, are in good health.	His father's death at a young age (from cardiac problems) may contribute to Mr. Pantelli's anxiety, although he may never talk about it. Explore this sensitive area when your patient teaching sessions begin.

Cardiac assessment

Taking your patient's medical history continued

Assessment information	Your written notes (sample)	Your mental notes (sample)
Review patient systems. Use the charts on the opposite page to conduct a physiologic investigation of your patient. They will help you to uncover signs and symptoms not already identified. Using words he can understand, ask your patient if he has any of the problems listed in the chart on the near right. If he does, record them and their possible causes. Also conduct a visual inspection using the chart on the far right as a guide. Record any signs of cardiac disease.	Patient has occasional headaches accompanied by pain behind his eyes, a possible symptom of stress. He denies any other problems. Patient has diagonal crease in his earlobes (McCarthy's sign), an indication of coronary artery disease.	Your McCarthy's sign finding adds further weight to a diagnosis of coronary artery disease.
Record patient personal and social history. To further assess your patient on a personal and social level, ask about: his job (how active and demanding it is); his diet (what he normally eats); his habits (how much alcohol, tobacco, coffee, and over-the-counter drugs he uses); and his activities (how much exercise he gets).	Mr. Pantelli states that, under normal circumstances, his job is not strenuous, but the store is temporarily understaffed and he's pitching in to help with the work. Usually, he eats a light breakfast, a quick lunch, and a big dinner meal. He enjoys traditional Italian foods that are heavily spiced and seasoned. He says that daily he drinks six cups of coffee and two beers. He also drinks a few glasses of wine each week. He takes aspirin and a bromide occasionally. He collects coins and enjoys fixing up their home, but says he doesn't get much exercise.	Note his diet. Later you can contact the hospital dietitian to suggest developing a diet that will allow Mr. Pantelli to eat some of the foods he likes after he returns home. Consider the possibility that Mr. Pantelli was taking bromides to treat angina pain, which he mistakenly thought was intestinal gas. When your patient teaching sessions begin, teach Mr. Pantelli how to differentiate types of chest pain.

Making a head-to-toe inspection

Hair: dry and brittle hair may indicate vascular insufficiency or some other heart disease

Ear: diagonal earlobe crease (McCarthy's sign) may indicate coronary artery disease

Head: subtle up and down movements in synchronization with heartbeat (Musset's sign) indicates aortic aneurysm or aortic insufficiency

Eyelids: yellow plaque (xanthelasma) may indicate elevated cholesterol

Eye: gray ring at junction if iris and sclera (corneal arcus) indicates hyperlipidemia

Lips and tongue: central cyanosis indicates oxygen deficiency (hypoxia), heart disease, and/or lung disease

Epigastric area: pulsations in aorta may indicate an abdominal aortic aneurysm

Upper right quadrant: pulsations in liver may indicate tricuspid regurgitation

Elbows: yellow plaque (xanthoma) may indicate elevated cholesterol

Skin color: pallor may indicate vasoconstriction; ruddiness may indicate polycythemia; cyanosis may indicate oxygen deficiency

Palms: pallor may indicate decreased hemoglobin count

Nailbeds: peripheral cyanosis indicates peripheral vascular disease and/or decreased cardiac output

Nails: clubbing indicates chronic hypoxemia and/or congenital heart disease; thickness indicates impaired oxygen delivery to extremities

Hair: absence or sparse growth may indicate poor peripheral circulation

Skin temperature: cool and dry skin indicates vascular insufficiency; cool and moist skin indicates vasoconstriction and/or anxiety

Lower leg: pretibial edema and pedal edema, with pitting, indicate congestive heart failure; without pitting, they may indicate vascular disease

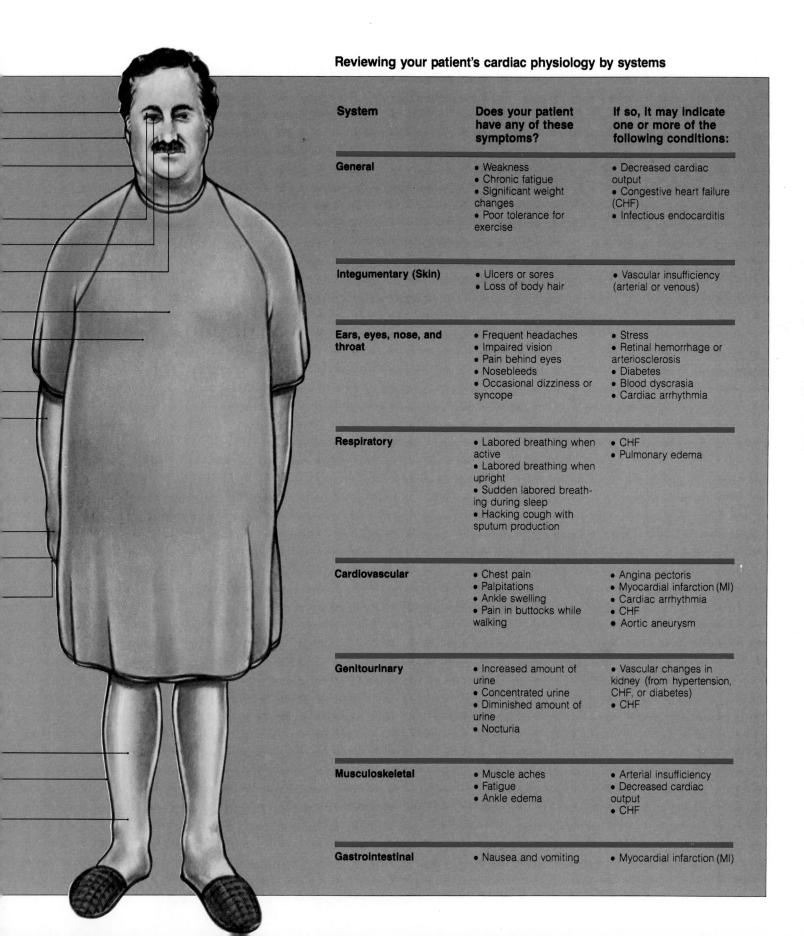

Reviewing your patient's cardiac physiology by systems

System	Does your patient have any of these symptoms?	If so, it may indicate one or more of the following conditions:
General	• Weakness • Chronic fatigue • Significant weight changes • Poor tolerance for exercise	• Decreased cardiac output • Congestive heart failure (CHF) • Infectious endocarditis
Integumentary (Skin)	• Ulcers or sores • Loss of body hair	• Vascular insufficiency (arterial or venous)
Ears, eyes, nose, and throat	• Frequent headaches • Impaired vision • Pain behind eyes • Nosebleeds • Occasional dizziness or syncope	• Stress • Retinal hemorrhage or arteriosclerosis • Diabetes • Blood dyscrasia • Cardiac arrhythmia
Respiratory	• Labored breathing when active • Labored breathing when upright • Sudden labored breathing during sleep • Hacking cough with sputum production	• CHF • Pulmonary edema
Cardiovascular	• Chest pain • Palpitations • Ankle swelling • Pain in buttocks while walking	• Angina pectoris • Myocardial infarction (MI) • Cardiac arrhythmia • CHF • Aortic aneurysm
Genitourinary	• Increased amount of urine • Concentrated urine • Diminished amount of urine • Nocturia	• Vascular changes in kidney (from hypertension, CHF, or diabetes) • CHF
Musculoskeletal	• Muscle aches • Fatigue • Ankle edema	• Arterial insufficiency • Decreased cardiac output • CHF
Gastrointestinal	• Nausea and vomiting	• Myocardial infarction (MI)

Cardiac assessment

Communicating with your patient

Do you understand exactly what your patient means when he talks to you? Does he understand you? Don't take such things for granted. Communicating effectively is easier said than done. Here are a few important points that will improve communication and help you compile a better cardiac assessment:

• Show concern. Since so much of a cardiac assessment is facts and figures, it's easy to appear clinical, cold, and remote to your patient. But the value of your assessment depends, in part, on the warmth and concern you project. The patient is affected by the image you convey. If you seem genuinely interested, you're more likely to develop rapport. The result is a broader, more perceptive record of his illness.

• Don't confuse the patient by using clinical terms. Instead, interview him by asking simple questions composed of easily understood words.

• Check his understanding by asking him to paraphrase your statement or questions. A misinterpreted question may get an incorrect answer. Also, repeat things he's said to you to make sure you understand him. Did he say what he meant to say? Don't rely solely on his ability to express himself for your data.

• Don't just listen to your patient. Watch him. His expressions and body language may tell you more than his words. For example, a distant or distracted expression may indicate that he doesn't understand.

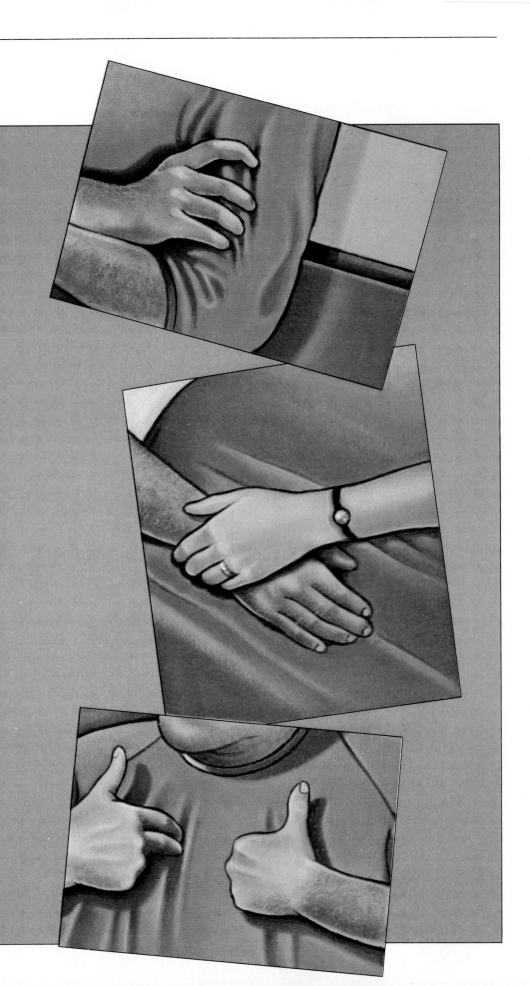

Assessing your patient's chest pain

Your patient complains of chest pain. Before you can help him, you have to find out what type of chest pain he's having. Once you learn the location, radiation, character, onset, and duration of the pain, you can relieve it. This chart will tell you how.

Type	Location and radiation	Character, onset, and duration	Precipitating events	Method of relief
Angina	• Substernal or retrosternal pain spreading across chest • May radiate to inside of either or both arms, the neck, or jaw	• Squeezing, heavy-pressure pain • Sudden onset • Usually subsides within 10 minutes	• Physical exertion • Hot, humid weather • Eating • Intense emotion	• Instruct patient to stop all physical activity • Administer nitrates sublingually, as ordered
Myocardial infarction	• Substernal or over precordium • May radiate throughout chest and arms to jaw	• Crushing, viselike pain • Sudden onset • More severe and prolonged than anginal pain	• Occurs spontaneously, often while resting (may be associated with dizziness, perspiration, nausea, and stress)	• Administer morphine, as ordered • Administer oxygen
Pericardial chest pain	• Substernal or left of sternum • May radiate to neck, arms, back, or epigastrium	• Sharp, intermittent pain (accentuated by swallowing, coughing, inspiration, or lying supine) • Severe, sudden onset • May occur intermittently over several days	• Upper respiratory infection • Myocardial infarction • Rheumatic fever • Pericarditis	• Instruct patient to bend forward • Administer analgesics • Administer oxygen, as needed
Pulmonary origin (pleuritis, pulmonary embolism [PE])	• Inferior portion of the pleura • May radiate to costal margins or upper abdomen	• Stabbing, knifelike pain (accentuated by respirations) • Sudden onset • May last a few days	• Anxiety (associated with coughing)	• Administer codeine for pain, as ordered • Administer antibiotic for infection, as ordered • Administer anti-coagulant for PE, as ordered
Esophageal pain	• Substernal • May radiate around chest to shoulders	• Burning, knotlike pain (simulating angina) • Sudden onset • Usually subsides within 15 to 20 minutes	• May occur spontaneously • Eating	• Administer antacids, as ordered • Instruct patient to sit up
Chest wall pain	• Costochondral or sternocostal junctions • Does not radiate	• Aching pain or soreness • Often begins as dull ache, increasing in intensity over a few days • Usually long-lasting	• Chest wall movement	• Apply heat • Administer muscle relaxants, as ordered • Doctor may inject a local anesthetic for pain, at affected junction
Anxiety	• Left chest (variable) • Does not radiate	• Sharp and stabbing pain, or vague discomfort • Sudden onset • May last less than a minute or for several days	• Fatigue (sometimes) • Intense emotion (sometimes)	• Administer sedatives, as ordered • Instruct patient to lie down, and breathe normally

Cardiac assessment

Learning basic assessment landmarks

To accurately inspect, palpate, percuss, and auscultate your patient's chest and heart—as well as document your findings—you first must know the location of several standard imaginary lines on the thorax. These lines or landmarks, shown in the drawing below, are called the midsternal line, right midclavicular line, and left midclavicular line.

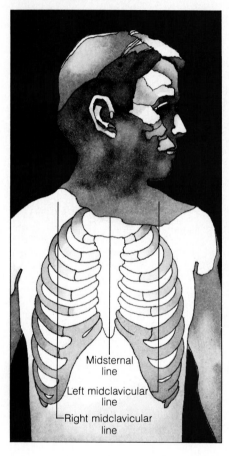

Midsternal line

Left midclavicular line

Right midclavicular line

Measuring arterial pulse

As you may know, your patient's arterial pulse reflects pressure changes in his left ventricle. This illustration shows you the major arteries you should palpate to measure arterial pulse: carotid, brachial, radial, femoral, popliteal, posterior tibial, and dorsalis pedis. Read the chart on the opposite page to help you evaluate the condition of the arterial wall, and the pulse rate, rhythm, and amplitude. You should take your patient's pulse for at least 1 minute. Here's the range you can expect, depending on your patient's age:

Age	Range
Under 1 month	90 to 170
Under 1 year	80 to 160
2 years	80 to 120
6 years	75 to 115
10 years	70 to 110
14 years	65 to 100
Over 14 years	60 to 100

To record your patient's pulse amplitude, use this standard scale:

0: pulse not palpable
+1: pulse is thready, weak, difficult to find, may fade in and out, and disappears easily with pressure.
+2: pulse is constant but not strong; light pressure must be applied or pulse will disappear.
+3: pulse considered normal. Is easily palpable, does not disappear with pressure.
+4: pulse is strong, bounding, and does not disappear with pressure.

Then, compare these measurements with those of the arteries that correspond bilaterally, and document your findings.

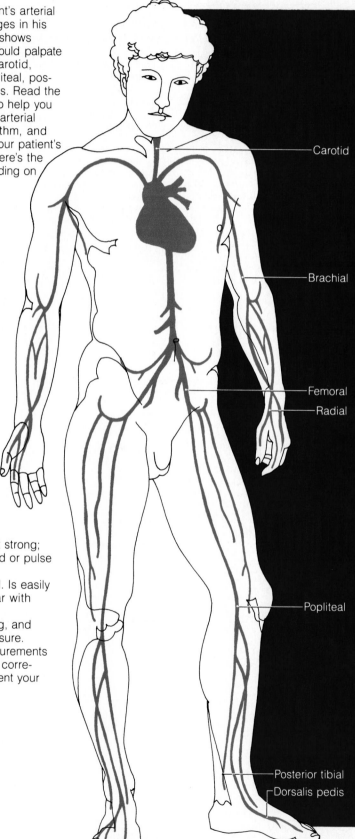

Carotid

Brachial

Femoral

Radial

Popliteal

Posterior tibial

Dorsalis pedis

What your patient's arterial pulse can tell you

Arterial wall
NORMAL CONDITION
- Soft and pliable

ABNORMAL CONDITION
- Tortuous and ropelike

POSSIBLE CAUSE OF ABNORMALITY
- Atherosclerosis

Rate
NORMAL CONDITION
- 60 to 100 beats per minute

ABNORMAL CONDITION
- Bradycardia (less than 60 beats per minute)
- Tachycardia (more than 100 beats per minute)
- Pulse deficit (peripheral and apical rates differ)

POSSIBLE CAUSE OF ABNORMALITY
- Sinus node disease, hypothyroidism
- Fever, hemorrhage, shock, anxiety
- Cardiac arrhythmia, atrial fibrillation

Rhythm
NORMAL CONDITION
- Regular

ABNORMAL CONDITION
- Irregular

POSSIBLE CAUSE OF ABNORMALITY
- Arrhythmias such as premature contractions or atrial fibrillation

Amplitude
NORMAL CONDITION
- Strong, easy to detect (+3)

ABNORMAL CONDITION
- Weak, faint, or not palpable
- Pulsus alternans (one weak beat/one strong beat)
- Pulsus paradoxus (change in amplitude during respiration)
- Plateau pulse (small amplitude, slow rise, sustained summit, gradual fill)
- Pulsus bisferiens (double beat at summit)
- Corrigan's, or water-hammer pulse (bounding, abrupt rise and fall back to diastolic level)

POSSIBLE CAUSE OF ABNORMALITY
- Partial occlusion of artery, heart disease, shock
- Left ventricular failure
- Severe lung disease, cardiac tamponade, advanced heart failure
- Aortic stenosis
- Aortic insufficiency

Equality of bilateral pulses
NORMAL CONDITION
- Equal

ABNORMAL CONDITION
- Unequal

POSSIBLE CAUSE OF ABNORMALITY
- Arterial obstructive disease, dissecting aneurysms

Measuring arterial blood pressure

When you take your patient's arterial blood pressure, you're measuring two things: the amount of pressure that the left ventricle exerts when it contracts (systolic reading), and the amount of pressure that the left ventricle exerts when it's at rest (diastolic reading). As you know, normal systolic pressure ranges from 100 to 140 mm Hg, and normal diastolic ranges from 60 to 90 mm Hg. To get an accurate reading, make sure you follow these precautions:
- Choose the correct cuff size. Its bladder should be one-fifth longer than the circumference of your patient's arm.
- Make sure the cuff you're using works properly.
- Avoid taking readings when your patient's blood pressure is abnormally high: for example, after meals, during or directly after exercise, during or immediately after an emotional upset, or just before or after he urinates or defecates.
- Place the cuff over his brachial artery.
- Deflate the cuff at the proper rate. If you deflate it too quickly, you won't have time to get an accurate reading. If you deflate it too slowly, you'll get a false high reading caused by venous congestion.
- Take two readings (one from each arm), with the patient standing, sitting, and lying down. His blood pressure should remain stable with each change in position. Here's the reading to expect, depending on your patient's age:

Age	Average reading
Under 1 year	63 mean (using flush technique)
2 years	96/30
4 years	98/60
6 years	105/60
10 years	112/64
Adolescent	120/75
Adult	130/80

What if your patient's blood pressure doesn't remain stable, and increases when he sits or reclines? Such changes may be caused by the patient's medication or indicate decreased cardiac output, incompetent valve action, cardiac tamponade, or constrictive pericarditis. Record your findings and notify doctor.

Assessing your patient's venous blood pressure

Assessing your patient's venous pressure is a simple but telling procedure. If your patient's venous pressure is elevated, he may have congestive heart failure, cardiac tamponade, or superior vena cava obstruction. You can judge your patient's venous blood pressure by inspecting his external and internal jugular veins.

Here's how. Seat your patient at a 45° angle. If his external jugular vein remains flat and barely visible above his clavicles, his venous pressure's normal. But, if the pulsations of his external jugular veins can be clearly seen 1½" (3.5 cm) above his sternal angle (where the clavicles meet), his venous pressure's abnormally high. In severe cases, jugular vein pulsations will be visible up to his jaw.

Next, attempt to observe internal jugular pulsations. To do this, you'll need tangential lighting. Angle the light source so that the internal jugular vein, which lies underneath the sternocleidomastoid muscle, casts a slight shadow. You can tell that his venous pressure's elevated if his internal jugular vein is prominent enough to cast a shadow as far as 1½" (3.5 cm) above his sternal angle. Document your observations.

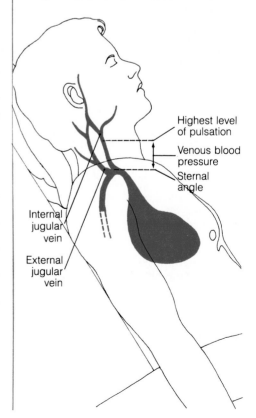

Highest level of pulsation

Venous blood pressure

Sternal angle

Internal jugular vein

External jugular vein

Cardiac assessment

Nurses' guide to breath sounds

This chart tells you four things: what you'll hear when you listen to your patient's breath sounds; where you'll hear them; where you *shouldn't* hear certain breath sounds; and what it indicates if you do.

Suppose you don't hear any of these breath sounds within their normal fields. Would you know what these findings indicate? Read this chart to find out.

Type	Description	Position in respiratory cycle	Normally heard over	Abnormally heard over
Vesicular	High-pitched and loud on inspiration; low-pitched and soft on expiration	More prominent during inspiration than during expiration	Peripheral lung fields	Peripheral lung fields in decreased volume; possibly indicating emphysema or pleural effusion
Bronchial or tracheal	High-pitched, loud, harsh, hollow	Less prominent during inspiration than during expiration	Trachea and the anterior of the mainstem bronchi	Peripheral lung fields; possibly indicating consolidation, as in pneumonia
Bronchovesicular	Moderate pitch and loudness	Equally prominent during inspiration and expiration	Major bronchi, upper anterior chest and posteriorly between scapulae	Peripheral lung fields; possibly an early indication of respiratory disease

Nurses' guide to adventitious sounds (rales, rhonchi, and rubs)

Types	Description	Position in respiratory cycle	Possible cause	Possible indication
Fine rales	High-pitched, crackling, and popping (like rubbing hairs between your fingers)	End of inspiration	Fluid in the smallest airways	Pneumonia or congestive heart failure (CHF)
Medium rales	Lower-pitched, louder, and wetter (like freshly opened bottle of carbonated soda)	Mid- to late inspiration or expiration	Fluid in the bronchioles	CHF, pneumonia, pulmonary edema, bronchitis, or emphysema
Coarse rales	Low-pitched and loud (like crushing cellophane between the fingers)	Inspiration and expiration	Fluid in the bronchi and trachea	Severe pulmonary edema
Sibilant rhonchi	High-pitched, musical, and squeaky (like whistling)	Predominant in expiration	Air passing through swollen small airways	Asthma or emphysema
Sonorous rhonchi	Lower-pitched and moaning (like snoring)	Throughout respiratory cycle, though predominantly heard during expiration. May clear with coughing.	Air passing through swollen large airways	Bronchitis, tracheobronchitis
Pleural rub	Coarse, grating, and low-pitched (like squeaking leather)	Throughout respiratory cycle, though loudest between inspiration and expiration.	Inflamed surfaces of pleurae rubbing together	Pleurisy, tuberculosis (TB), pulmonary infection, pneumonia, or cancer

Examining your patient's thorax and lungs

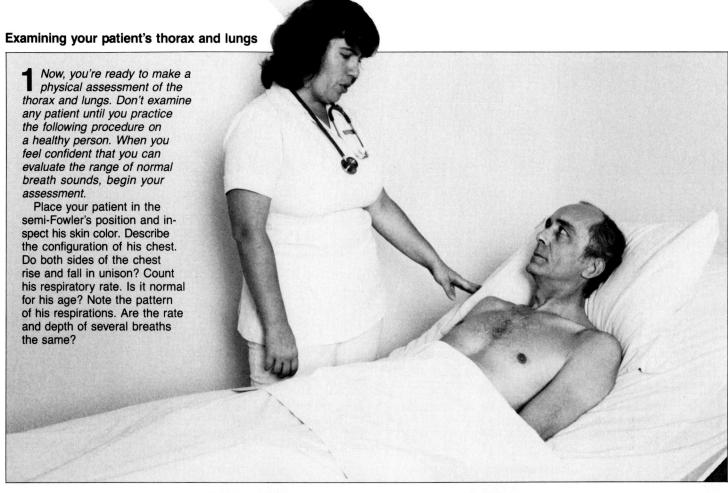

1 *Now, you're ready to make a physical assessment of the thorax and lungs. Don't examine any patient until you practice the following procedure on a healthy person. When you feel confident that you can evaluate the range of normal breath sounds, begin your assessment.*

Place your patient in the semi-Fowler's position and inspect his skin color. Describe the configuration of his chest. Do both sides of the chest rise and fall in unison? Count his respiratory rate. Is it normal for his age? Note the pattern of his respirations. Are the rate and depth of several breaths the same?

2 Next, palpate the patient's chest to determine the positions of the thorax and lungs. Does he have any chest wall abnormalities? Does he complain of pain as you palpate? Can you feel vibrations throughout his chest as he breathes? Record your findings.

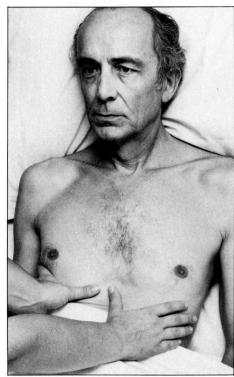

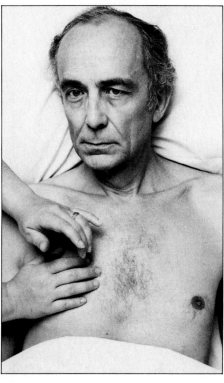

3 Now, percuss your patient's chest for any audible abnormalities. When you percuss over the lungs (which are air-filled structures), you should hear a resonant sound. When you percuss over the heart (a fluid-filled structure), your percussion should produce a dull sound. When you percuss over bone (a solid structure), you should get a flat sound. When you percuss a large cavity, such as the stomach, you should hear a tympanic sound. If you don't hear the expected type of percussing sound, suspect something's wrong and record your findings for further investigation.

Cardiac assessment

Examining your patient's thorax and lungs continued

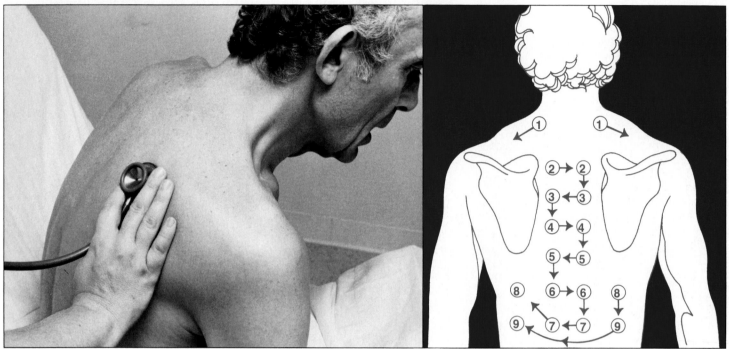

4 Finally, auscultate your patient to evaluate normal breath sounds and detect abnormal or adventitious ones. Begin by instructing him to breathe quietly through his mouth, a little more deeply than usual. Warm the diaphragm side of your stethoscope. Then place it firmly on your patient's back. Follow the listening pattern indicated by the arrows on this illustration and compare each side as you move downward. Record your findings, using the charts on page 16 as your guide.

5 Then, on your patient's anterior chest, listen from above his clavicles to the sixth rib, following the arrows shown here.

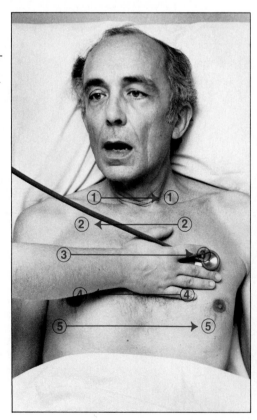

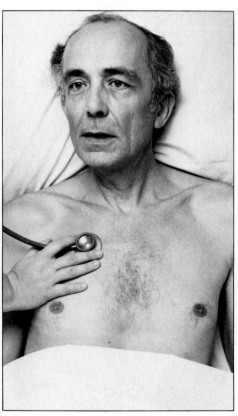

6 Finally, ask your patient to say the number 99. Listen with your stethoscope. If the sound of his voice is muffled and indistinct, transmission is normal. But if the sound of his voice is loud and distinct, he may be suffering from congestion or fluid build-up.

Document all your findings in your nurses' notes.

For full details on how to examine the thorax, see the NURSING PHOTOBOOK volumes, *Providing Respiratory Care* and *Assessing Your Patients*.

Inspection and palpation areas

The illustration below shows the six areas where you'll inspect and palpate cardiac activity. They're named for the structures you'll palpate underneath the chest wall. Here are their names and locations:
• Sternoclavicular area: located just above the top of the sternum at the junction of the clavicles.
• Aortic area: located just above the aortic valve in the 2nd intercostal space on the right sternal border.
• Pulmonic area: located just above the pulmonic valve in the 2nd intercostal space on the left sternal border.
• Right ventricular area: located just above the right ventricle where the 5th rib joins the left sternal border.
• Left ventricular area: located just above the left ventricle, which is left of the sternum at the 5th intercostal space to the right of the midclavicular line.
• Epigastric area: located just above the epigastric area, which is at the base of the sternum between the cartilage of the left and right 7th ribs.

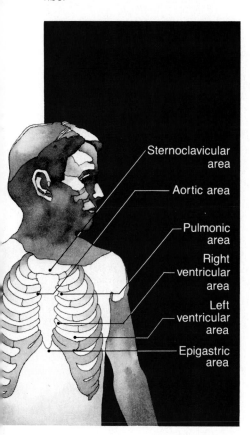

Sternoclavicular area
Aortic area
Pulmonic area
Right ventricular area
Left ventricular area
Epigastric area

Inspecting and palpating your patient's heart

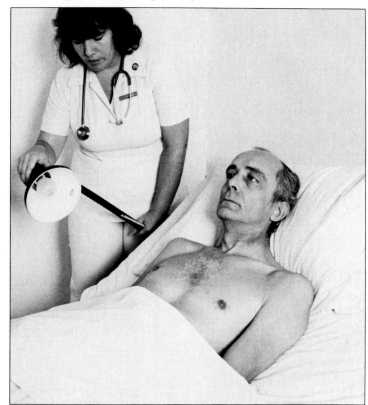

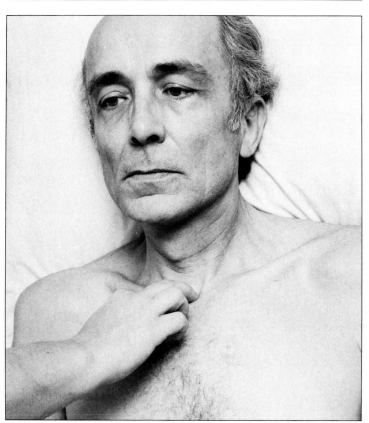

1 Now you're ready to make a physical assessment of your patient's heart. This includes inspection and palpation, as outlined here, and percussion and auscultation, which we'll explain later.
Begin by explaining the procedure to the patient. Seat him upright at a 45° angle. Place a light source level with his chest so that movement of his chest wall casts a slight shadow. Visualize where his heart's located beneath his chest wall and observe that area. If you spot a localized heaving or lifting of his chest wall, this may indicate cardiac hypertrophy. Record your observations.

2 To palpate the heart, you'll either use the heel of your hand (for large areas) or the tips of your fingers (for small areas). Usually you'll have the greatest sensitivity using light pressure, but if your patient has a fat or muscular chest, you'll have to apply more pressure.
Nursing tip: Warm your hands before touching your patient to help him relax and make palpation easier.
Begin palpation at the sternoclavicular area, using the illustration on the left as your guide to the correct sites. Be especially alert in the sternoclavicular area for strong pulsations. They may indicate an aortic aneurysm.

Cardiac assessment

Inspecting and palpating your patient's heart continued

3 Now, palpate the aortic area. Here you may feel thrills, in addition to sharp pulsations. A thrill is a rapid vibration beneath the skin that feels like water running through a hose or a cat purring. Thrills indicate valvular stenosis.

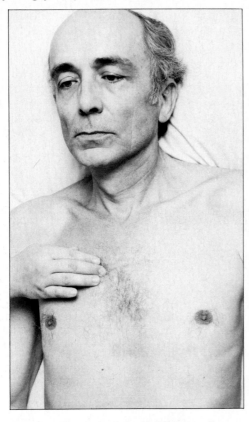

5 Now, palpate the right ventricular area, staying alert for thrills or heaves, as described before.

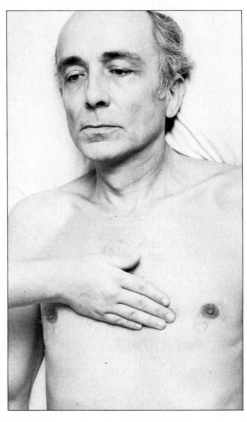

4 Palpate the pulmonic area next, as the nurse is doing here. You may feel strong pulsations or thrills in this area, too.

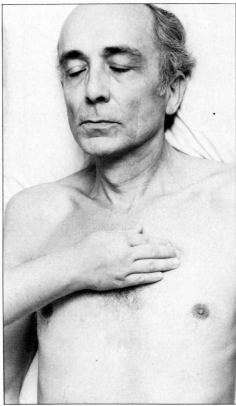

6 Next, palpate the left ventricular area. This area is also called the point of maximum impulse (PMI). Note the impulse's amplitude, size, intensity, location, and duration. If all's well, you'll feel a light impulse in an area about ¾" in diameter on the left midclavicular line. In such cases, the impulse will begin at the time of the first heart sound, then continue through the first half of systole. Note any extra impulses. If the PMI is to the left of the left midclavicular line, suspect ventricular enlargement or failure.

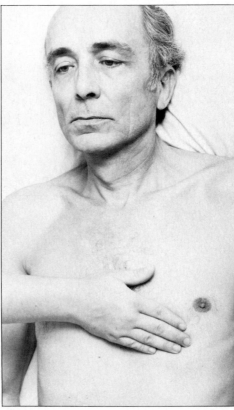

What your inspection and palpation findings mean

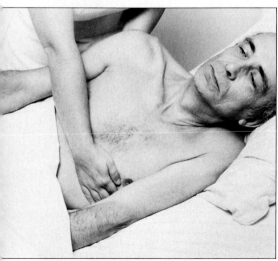

7 Palpate the epigastric area. To do this, tuck your fingertips under the rim of your patient's rib cage at the sternum. You should be able to feel the aorta pulsating against your fingertips and the right ventricle beating against the side of your fingers. If you feel an abnormally strong pulsation, suspect an aortic aneurysm.

8 Finally, turn your patient so he's in the left lateral position. This new position may reveal thrills or heaves that are hard to palpate because they're not near the skin surface. Palpate the right and left ventricular areas in particular. Then, record all of your findings and document the procedure.

Inspection and palpation area	Possible observations	Possible abnormalities
Sternoclavicular	• Abnormally strong pulsation	• Aortic aneurysm
Aortic	• Abnormally abrupt pulsation	• Rheumatic heart disease • Systemic hypertension
	• Thrill	• Aortic stenosis
Pulmonary	• Abnormally abrupt pulsation	• Essential pulmonary hypertension
	• Thrill	• Pulmonic stenosis
	• Abnormally strong or forceful pulsation	• Emphysema, mitral stenosis • Extensive pneumonia • Pulmonary embolism
Right ventricular	• Thrill	• Ventricular septal defect
	• Heave and lift with each heartbeat	• Right ventricular hypertrophy • Pulmonic stenosis • Systemic hypertension • Emphysema, mitral stenosis • Extensive pneumonia
Left ventricular	• Thrill	• Mitral stenosis
	• Gallop	• Ischemia • Injury • Myocardial infarction
	• Impulse far to the left or low	• Aortic regurgitation • Aortic stenosis • Left ventricular hypertrophy • Systemic hypertension
	• Impulse covering a large area	• Aortic regurgitation • Aortic stenosis • Left ventricular hypertrophy • Systemic hypertension
	• Impulse long in duration and/or abnormally strong	• Aortic regurgitation • Aortic stenosis • Left ventricular hypertrophy • Systemic hypertension
Epigastric	• Abnormally strong pulsation	• Aortic aneurysm

Cardiac assessment

Percussing your patient's heart

You'll percuss your patient's chest to get an idea of the size and location of his heart. Normally, you'll find the heart's left sternal border on the left midclavicular line, at the 5th intercostal space. Begin percussing the area just to the patient's left of this landmark and move across his chest. When the percussion sound changes from resonant (lung tissue) to dull (heart tissue), you have reached the left cardiac border. Continue to percuss the left border until you can visualize the position of the entire left border.

Since the right border of the heart lies underneath the bone of the sternum, you can't percuss it as you did the left border. But, you can learn if the right ventricle's enlarged. Here's how:

Percuss the sternum, identifying the flat sound that means you're directly over bone. If, as you move down the sternum, you begin hearing dull sounds instead, suspect an enlarged right ventricle. Your findings can be confirmed by a chest X-ray.

Record all your observations during this procedure and document them in your nurses' notes.

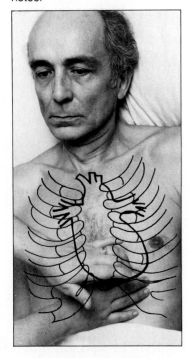

Cardiac auscultation areas

This illustration shows the four areas where you'll auscultate the heart. They're named after the valves whose function you'll be evaluating when you auscultate.
• Aortic area: located at the 2nd intercostal space, right sternal border
• Pulmonic area: located at the 2nd intercostal space, left sternal border
• Tricuspid area: located at the 5th intercostal space, left sternal border
• Mitral area: located at the 5th intercostal space, left midclavicular line.

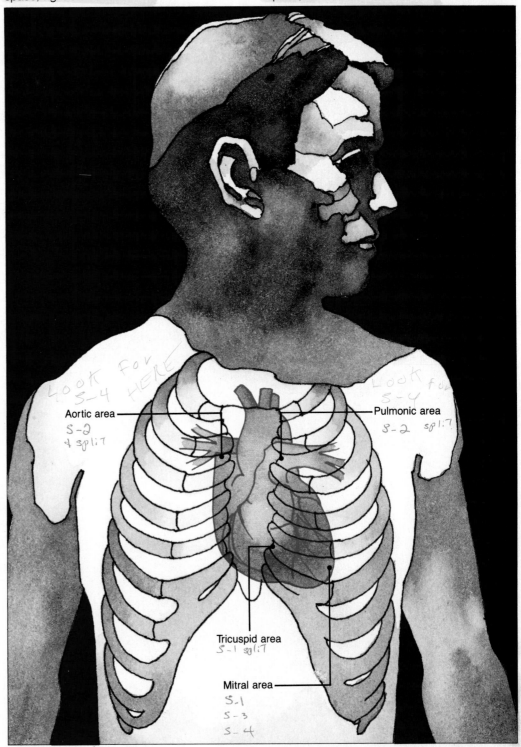

Aortic area

Pulmonic area

Tricuspid area

Mitral area

Nurses' guide to heart sounds

What can you expect to hear when you auscultate the heart? This chart tells you. Study it carefully to learn about normal and abnormal heart sounds.

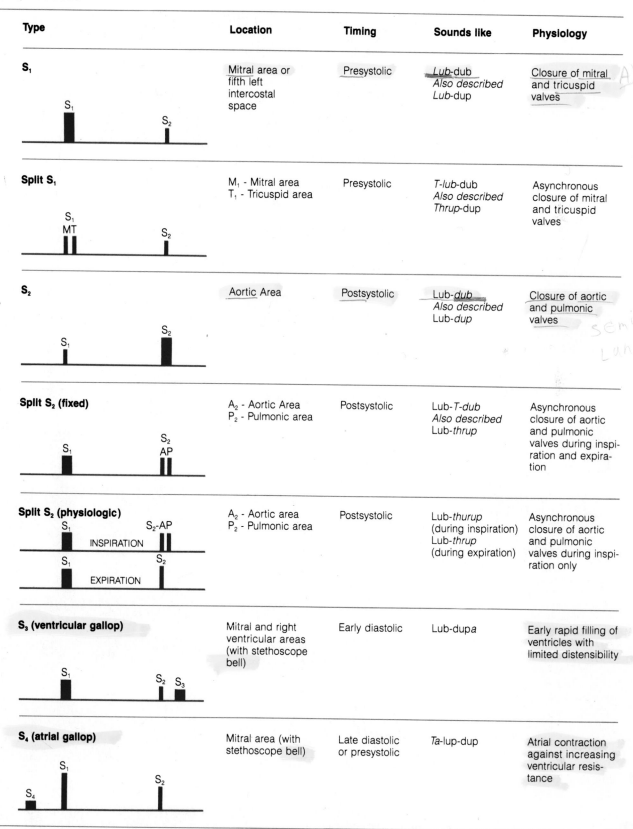

Type	Location	Timing	Sounds like	Physiology
S₁	Mitral area or fifth left intercostal space	Presystolic	*Lub*-dub *Also described* *Lub*-dup	Closure of mitral and tricuspid valves
Split S₁	M₁ - Mitral area T₁ - Tricuspid area	Presystolic	*T-lub*-dub *Also described* *Thrup*-dup	Asynchronous closure of mitral and tricuspid valves
S₂	Aortic Area	Postsystolic	Lub-*dub* *Also described* Lub-*dup*	Closure of aortic and pulmonic valves
Split S₂ (fixed)	A₂ - Aortic Area P₂ - Pulmonic area	Postsystolic	Lub-*T-dub* *Also described* Lub-*thrup*	Asynchronous closure of aortic and pulmonic valves during inspiration and expiration
Split S₂ (physiologic)	A₂ - Aortic area P₂ - Pulmonic area	Postsystolic	Lub-*thurup* (during inspiration) Lub-*thrup* (during expiration)	Asynchronous closure of aortic and pulmonic valves during inspiration only
S₃ (ventricular gallop)	Mitral and right ventricular areas (with stethoscope bell)	Early diastolic	Lub-dup*a*	Early rapid filling of ventricles with limited distensibility
S₄ (atrial gallop)	Mitral area (with stethoscope bell)	Late diastolic or presystolic	*Ta*-lup-dup	Atrial contraction against increasing ventricular resistance

Cardiac assessment

Learning about heart murmurs

When you listen for heart sounds, you may hear more than the sounds identified as S_1 through S_4. If they're not merely accidental sounds, like coughing or hiccuping, then you may be listening to a murmur. You'll hear a murmur, or audible vibration, when blood flow's obstructed or abnormal. The four illustrations here show the various abnormalities possible. Familiarize yourself with the following terms used in identifying murmurs. Then, study the chart on the opposite page to learn about the different types of murmurs:

• *Timing:* You'll identify the murmur by its occurrence in the systolic or diastolic phase. You'll find an early systolic murmur is usually called an ejection murmur and a murmur heard throughout systole is called a pansystolic or holosystolic murmur.

• *Quality:* Describe the quality or sound of the murmur as blowing, harsh, musical, or rumbling.

• *Pitch:* Identify the pitch or frequency of the murmur as high or low.

• *Location:* Name the auscultation location where you hear the murmur best: aortic, pulmonic, tricuspid, or mitral.

• *Radiation:* List the bordering structures in which the murmur also is heard.

• *Loudness:* Employ this rating system to describe the volume of the murmur: 1 - barely heard; 2 - faint but distinct; 3 - moderately detectable; 4 - loud; 5 - very loud; 6 - heard before stethoscope comes in contact with the chest.

• *Intensity:* Decide in which part of the respiration cycle the murmur is more distinct. If more distinct on inspiration, describe it as crescendo. If more distinct on expiration, call it decrescendo. If equally distinct throughout the cycle, describe it as crescendo-decrescendo.

Unlike the other terms, intensity and loudness vary depending on the patient, so these listings are not included in the chart on the opposite page.

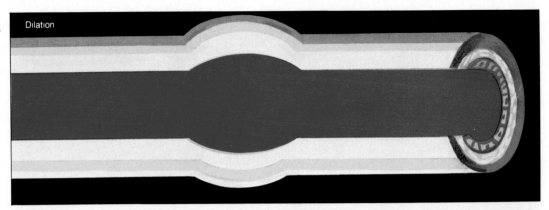

Dilation

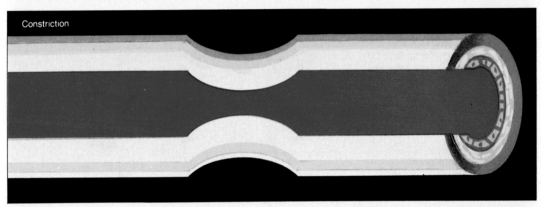

Constriction

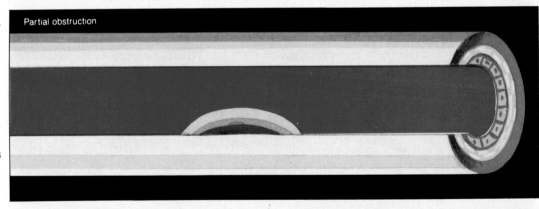

Partial obstruction

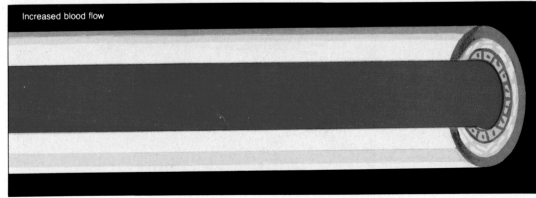

Increased blood flow

Learning about heart murmurs continued

Timing	Quality	Pitch	Location	Radiation	Condition
Systolic ejection	Harsh, rough	Medium to high	Pulmonic	Toward left shoulder and neck	Pulmonary stenosis
Midsystolic	Harsh, rough	Medium to high	Aortic and supra-sternal notch	Toward carotid arteries or apex	Aortic stenosis
	Harsh	High	Tricuspid	Precordium	Ventricular septal defect
Holosystolic	Blowing	High	Mitral, lower left sternal border	Toward left axilla	Mitral insufficiency
	Blowing	High	Tricuspid	Toward apex	Tricuspid insufficiency
Early diastolic	Blowing	High	Midleft sternal edge (not aortic area)	Toward sternum	Aortic insufficiency
	Blowing	High	Pulmonic	Toward sternum	Pulmonary insufficiency
Mid- to late diastolic	Rumbling	Low	Mitral	Usually none	Mitral stenosis
	Rumbling	Low	Tricuspid, lower sternal border	Usually none	Tricuspid stenosis

Learning about clicks and snaps

The systolic click and opening snap are other abnormal sounds you may hear when listening to your patient's heart. The click can occur at any time during the systolic phase of the cardiac cycle. Exactly when you hear it determines what the click is called. Opening snaps, on the other hand, can occur only when the heart is in diastole. This chart tells you more.

Type of sound	Timing	Location	Possible indications
Ejection click	Onset of systolic ejection	Aortic area, with patient in left lateral position	Aortic stenosis, aortic insufficiency, coarctation of the aorta, aneurysms of the ascending aorta, hypertension with aortic dilation
		Pulmonic area, with patient in left lateral position	Pulmonic stenosis, pulmonary hypertension
Non-ejection click	Mid- to late systole	Mitral area, with patient in left lateral position	Prolapsed mitral valve syndrome
Opening snap	Early diastole	4th intercostal space, at left sternal border	Mitral stenosis
		2nd intercostal space, at right sternal border	Tricuspid stenosis

Cardiac assessment

Auscultating your patient's heart

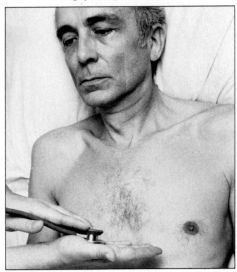

1 *The final step of cardiac assessment is auscultating your patient's heart. You'll do this to assess his heart sounds.*

Begin by explaining what you're going to do. Then, seat your patient at a 45° angle. Warm the stethoscope's bell and diaphragm between your hands so the patient won't tense up when you place it on his chest.

2 Place the stethoscope's diaphragm over your patient's aortic area. To locate the area's exact position, find the second right intercostal space, near the sternal border. (Use the illustration on page 24 as your guide to locating all the sites discussed in this photostory.)

If all's well, you should hear normal heart sounds S_1 and S_2 (lub-dub). S_2 will be louder in this area. Note the pitch, intensity, duration, and quality of each sound.

☎ *Nursing tip:* Don't try to listen to both heart sounds at once. Distinguish the S_1 sound and listen to it for several beats. Then, do the same for the S_2 sound.

Next, listen for the systolic and diastolic intervals. The systolic interval is the pause between S_1 and S_2 (lub-dub). The diastolic interval is the longer pause between S_2 and S_1 (dub-lub).

Count your patient's heartbeats for a minute, noting rate and rhythm. If you hear an irregular rhythm, describe its irregularity. Is it irregular in a pattern or is it chaotic? If it's a frequent or constant irregularity, notify the doctor. He may order an electrocardiogram (EKG).

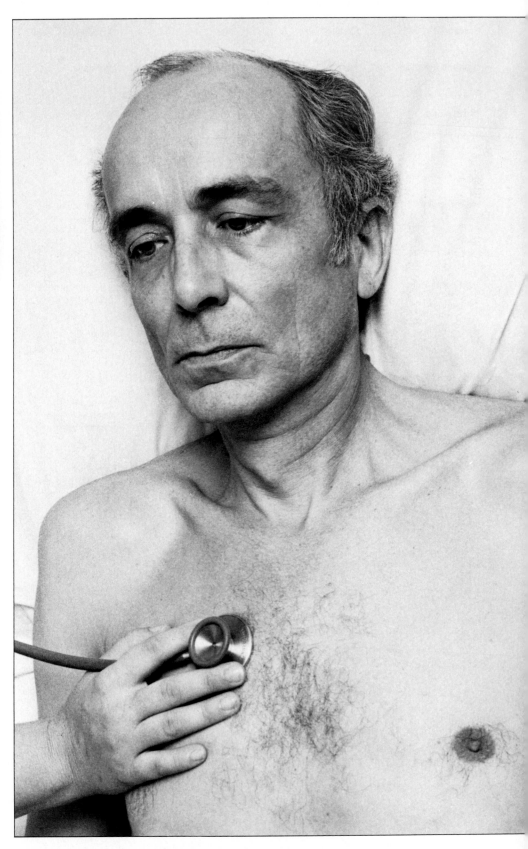

3 Now, using the stethoscope's bell, listen over the aortic area for low-frequency sounds (S_3 and S_4), murmurs, clicks, and rubs. If you have difficulty distinguishing S_3 and S_4, remember their timing in the cardiac cycle: S_3 occurs early in the diastolic interval; S_4 occurs prior to the systolic interval. If you still have difficulty distinguishing them, you'll probably have better luck later listening over the mitral area, where they can be heard more clearly.

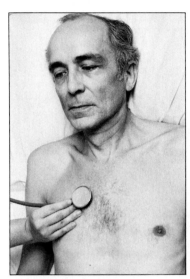

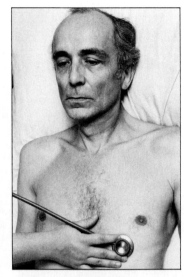

6 Once again, repeat this assessment procedure in the mitral area (fifth intercostal space, left midclavicular line). Here, you can expect S_1 to sound louder than S_2.

4 Repeat all of steps 2 and 3 over the pulmonic area of the heart (second intercostal space, left sternal border). Note the pitch, intensity, duration, and quality of the heart sounds. Since in this area S_2 is louder than S_1, listen in particular for split S_2 (fixed or physiologic). Then, count your patient's heartbeat for a minute, noting rate and rhythm. Also, check for S_3 and S_4 sounds, murmurs, clicks, and rubs.

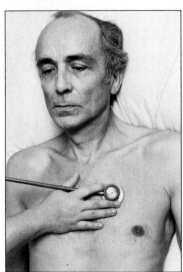

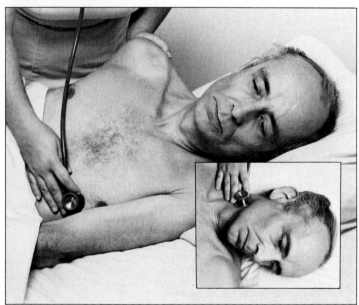

5 Repeat this assessment procedure in the tricuspid area (fifth intercostal space, left sternal border). Here, you'll find S_1 sounds louder than S_2.

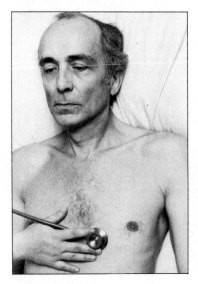

7 Now, turn your patient so he's in the left lateral position, as shown here. Auscultate his heart again. This position will help you hear hard-to-detect murmurs and other abnormalities. Don't be surprised if the murmurs fade in and out. Describe exactly what you hear.

▣ *Nursing tip:* As you gain more experience examining the heart, you can palpate and auscultate the patient in the sitting position and then palpate and auscultate his heart in the left lateral position. This way, you won't have to turn him so much.

[Inset] Finally, listen over your patient's carotid arteries for bruits (whooshing sounds) that have radiated from the heart. To do this, have the patient turn his head away from the side you plan to listen to. Then, as you hold your stethoscope gently over the artery, instruct the patient to hold his breath. Repeat the procedure on the other side of his neck. Then, listen over his abdominal aorta for bruits. If you hear any, suspect an aortic aneurysm.

Record all you've heard. Document the entire procedure in your nurses' notes.

Cardiac assessment

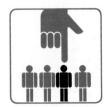

Assessing the pediatric patient

To assess a pediatric patient physically, use the same method you use on an adult. But, observe the following variations:

• *Blood pressure reading:* The diastolic sound you hear in an infant or child won't be as distinct as an adult's.

If you can't hear either the diastolic or systolic sounds, which frequently happens with patients under age one, use the flush technique instead. To do this, elevate the infant's arm or thigh (either's OK, since the arm and thigh pressure of those under age one are equal). Wait until the skin blanches. Now, apply the proper size cuff to the infant and inflate it to about 75 mm Hg. Then, lower the limb and begin deflating the cuff. Note the pressure reading when the entire limb flushes with color. This approximate reading is the *infant's mean blood pressure.*

A pediatric patient's *pulse pressure* (the difference between systolic and diastolic readings) is 20 to 50 mm Hg throughout childhood. If it's less than 20 mm Hg, the patient may have aortic stenosis. If the pulse pressure's more than 50 mm Hg—and you used the proper size pressure cuff—your patient may have patent ductus arteriosis or aortic regurgitation.

• *Arterial palpation:* You may not be able to locate your patient's popliteal pulse. Or, you may not be able to locate the post-tibial or dorsalis pedis pulse. For pulses that can be palpated, their rate fluctuates rapidly.

Important: When you palpate radial and femoral pulses, expect them to beat synchronously. If they don't, suspect coarctation of the aorta.

• *Chest inspection:* The normal infant and young child exhibit what is called diaphragmatic breathing, and show minimal thoracic activity. So, you'll assess the pattern of their breathing by observing their abdomens, not their chests. This pattern changes with aging. You'll assess the breathing patterns of older children in the same way you assess an adult's—by observing the chest.

• *Chest percussion:* Percuss the pediatric patient very lightly. If you hear hyperresonance over the left side of his chest, don't automatically assume this indicates a pneumothorax. It may only indicate he has air bubbles in his stomach.

• *Chest auscultation:* Don't be discouraged if you can't immediately differentiate between heart sounds S_1 and S_2. At first, you may also have trouble identifying heart sounds and lung sounds because your area for auscultation is so small. However, rest assured both skills can be acquired with practice.

You may hear coarse sounds in the patient's chest. Don't be alarmed. Such sounds may only indicate mucus in his trachea. If you hear a sinus arrhythmia in a child, instruct him to hold his breath. This should make the arrhythmia disappear. If you hear a sinus arrhythmia in an infant, observe his respirations as you listen to his heart. The arrhythmia will speed up with inspiration and slow down with expiration.

Identifying common congenital heart defects

How frequently will you encounter a congenital heart defect in a newborn infant? Only about 5 times in every 1,000 births. But for those 5 infants, your skill in recognizing that defect may mean the difference between life and death. What should you look for? Stay alert for the following signs and report them to the doctor immediately:

• *Difficulty breathing,* evidenced by rapid, shallow respirations, flaring nostrils, rib retractions, and expiratory grunting. This is especially noticeable during feedings or when infant is crying. Observe sleeping infant closely for tachypnea.

• *Increasing pulse rate,* especially in resting infant.

• *Failure to thrive.* Infant does not gain weight satisfactorily.

• *Cyanosis.* Bluish tinge noticeable on infant's heels, lips, and fingernails. (On dark-skinned infants, look for cyanosis on mucous membranes.) Always use direct lighting or you may miss early signs.

• *Swollen eyelids and face.* An early sign of right-sided heart failure.

• *Recurrent respiratory infection.* A child with a previously undiagnosed heart defect may have a history of recurring respiratory infections.

Remember, the type of heart defect and its severity determine the signs and symptoms. In some cases, clinical evidence of a heart defect may not be found until the patient reaches childhood.

Surgical repair of a defect may be immediate or delayed, depending on the infant's condition and the size and type of the defect. For more details on the types of heart defects and their clinical pictures, study the following pages.

AORTIC STENOSIS
Narrowing of the aortic valve.

Circulatory effects
• To maintain aortic pressure, left ventricle pressure increases, causing left ventricular hypertrophy.

Clinical picture
• Systolic ejection murmur is atypical.
• Infant may have intractable congestive heart failure, dyspnea, hypotension, tachycardia, rales, and cyanosis.

PULMONARY STENOSIS
Narrowing of the pulmonic valve, as shown in this illustration. Note: Infants may also have narrowing of the pulmonary artery, which is not shown here.

Circulatory effects
• Right ventricular pressure increases to overcome obstruction.

Clinical picture
• Midsystolic ejection murmur is prominent. Thrill heard in second left intercostal space.
• Infant is normal in weight, growth, and development, unless defect is severe. He may experience dyspnea, fatigue, peripheral cyanosis, and cold extremities.

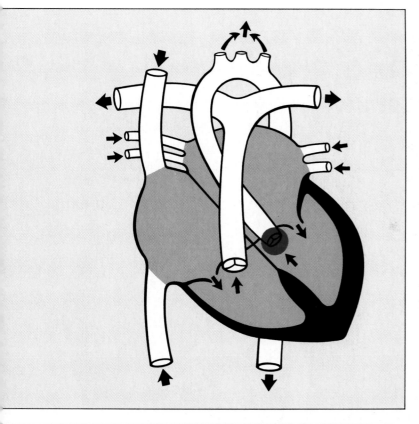

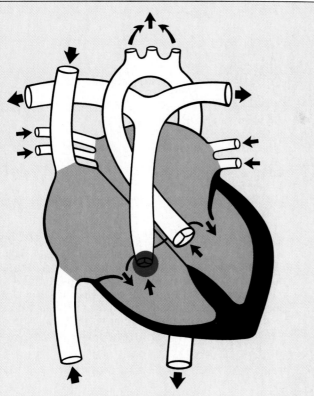

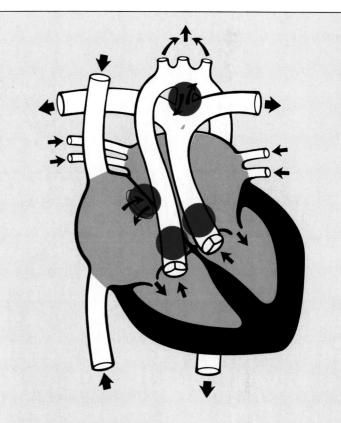

TRANSPOSITION OF GREAT VESSELS
Aorta leaves right ventricle; pulmonary artery leaves left ventricle. Usually associated with ventricular septal defect, atrial septal defect, or patent ductus arteriosus.

Circulatory effects
• Unoxygenated blood flows through right atrium and ventricle and out aorta to systemic circulation.
• Oxygenated blood flows from lungs to left atrium and ventricle and out pulmonary artery to lungs.

Clinical picture
• Predominant signs and symptoms shortly after birth are those of congestive heart failure (CHF), severe cyanosis, and extreme dyspnea.
• Systolic murmur heard if ventricular septal defect (VSD) is present.
• Sucking reflex poor.

Cardiac assessment

Identifying common congenital heart defects continued

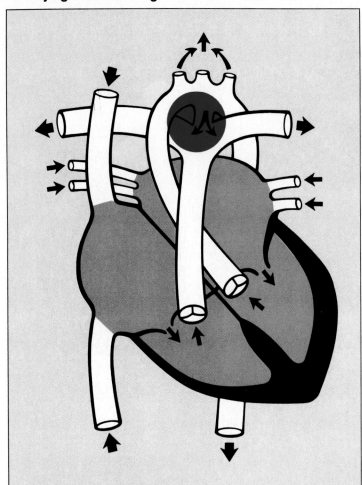

PATENT DUCTUS ARTERIOSUS (PDA)
Opening between the descending aorta and bifurcation of the pulmonary artery

Circulatory effects
• Acyanotic defect
• Left to right shunt may cause pulmonary artery hypertension.
• Pulse pressure may be widened; pulses full or bounding.

Clinical picture
• Continuous murmur with machinelike sound may be only sign of defect. Murmur loudest at left upper sternal border and under clavicle.
• Increased incidence in premature infants
• Infant may show signs of CHF if defect's severe.
• Bounding posterior tibial, dorsalis pedis, and palmar pulses; dyspnea on exertion; and vigorous precordial movements.

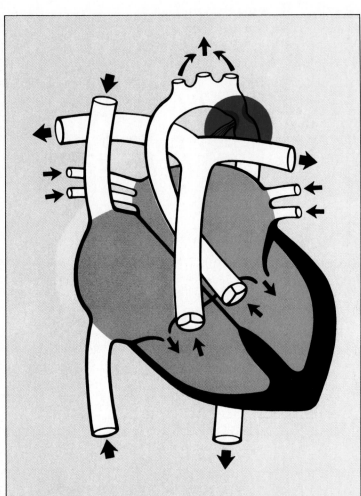

COARCTATION OF THE AORTA
Constriction of descending aorta near the ductus arteriosus

Circulatory effects
• Acyanotic defect
• Elevated blood pressures in ascending aorta and left ventricle
• Insufficient mitral valve
• Pulmonary hypertension
• Aneurysms and/or increased blood pressure in upper extremities.

Clinical picture
• Murmur is systolic ejection click heard at base and apex of heart. Associated with systolic or continuous murmur between scapulae. Pulses in upper extremities are full. Pulses in lower extremities are weak or absent.
• Because of the pressure differences in infant's upper and lower body, he may have dizziness, headaches, fainting, nosebleeds, leg cramping, and cold feet.

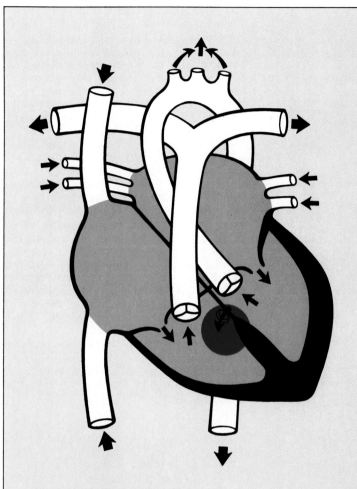

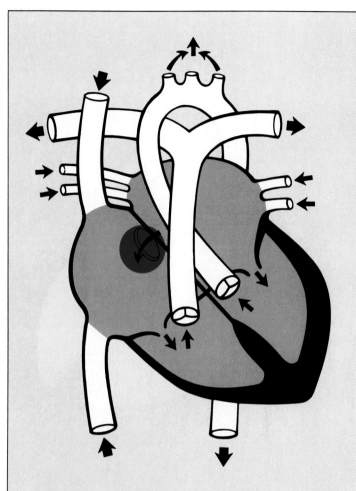

VENTRICULAR SEPTAL DEFECT (VSD)
One or more openings between the ventricles

Circulatory effects
• Acyanotic defect
• Blood flows from area of higher concentration to area of lower concentration.
• This left-to-right shunt may cause pulmonary congestion and pulmonary artery hypertension.

Clinical picture
• Murmur may be only sign of defect. Harsh, systolic sound heard in left lower sternal border, associated with palpable thrill.
• Patient may show signs of CHF, if defect is severe.

ATRIAL SEPTAL DEFECT (ASD)
One or more openings between the atria; includes ostium secundum, ostium primum, and sinus venosus.

Circulatory effects
• Acyanotic defect
• Left-to-right shunt may cause pulmonary artery hypertension.
• Atrial arrhythmias secondary to right atrial overload and resultant interference with conduction system.

Clinical picture
• Murmur may be only sign of defect. Soft, pulmonic systolic ejection is greatest in second and third left intercostal spaces.
• Infant is usually acyanotic but may develop cyanosis.
• If defect is severe, patient may develop CHF in late childhood.

Cardiac assessment

Identifying common congenital heart defects continued

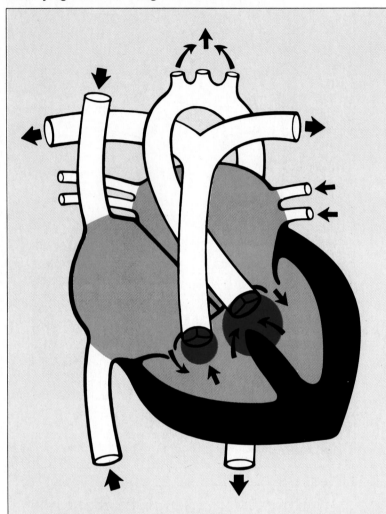

TETRALOGY OF FALLOT
Four defects: ventricular septal defect (VSD); overriding aorta; pulmonary stenosis; and right ventricular hypertrophy

Circulatory effects
• Pulmonary stenosis restricts blood flow to lungs.
• Unoxygenated blood is shunted through the VSD.
• Oxygenated and unoxygenated blood is mixed in the left ventricle and pumped out the aorta.

Clinical picture
• Single S_2 systolic murmur loudest in second and third inter-costal spaces at left sternal border.
• Infant has intense cyanosis, severe dyspnea on exertion, and limpness. If untreated, may be fatal. Compensating squatting position common in child.

Helping the cardiac patient's family

Everyone knows the patient with a cardiac problem needs special attention. But, don't forget that his family and friends need help, too. The heart, physiologically, is the center of life. This fact alone makes family and friends of the cardiac patient acutely concerned. When you consider that many people also attribute some very special emotions to the heart, such as love and despair, your support and guidance are essential.

Perhaps the most important service you can provide to family and friends is to act as their information resource. Consider the case of Mrs. Carolyn Vincent. Her husband has suffered a myocardial infarction. After a hectic rush of events, she finds herself suddenly alone, disoriented, and afraid, outside the doors of the CCU. People in white bustle past without speaking to her. She feels ignored, not know-ing these people are lab technicians, dietitians, and EKG technicians just going about their jobs. Suddenly, a group of medical students enters the CCU. She becomes alarmed, thinking that all those doctors are needed to treat her husband.

Show compassion for Mrs. Vincent. Introduce yourself. Just a few minutes of your time to talk and answer questions can calm her. Provide the following information:
• location of husband
• his condition
• health-care professionals in attendance
• procedures being used to relieve his problem.

In addition, assure her that you'll let her know as soon as possible when she can see him. Promise to keep her informed and find her a place to sit.

Parents of newborn infants with congenital heart defects face a special challenge: ac-cepting the fact that *their* new child has a defect. To help them cope, you need to be sensitive to their feelings and show compassion for their sense of loss. Listen closely to what they're saying to discover exactly how to help. Maybe they don't really understand what's wrong with their child. Do your best to clear up their misconceptions. Perhaps they feel guilty and blame themselves in some way for their child's defect. Assure them that nothing they did (or didn't do) caused the defect. If you sense they need spiritual help, you could offer to call their pastor, priest, or rabbi.

Examine your own feelings, too. In cases of personal grief, you may find yourself pulling away emotionally to attend to your own sorrow. But don't act remote. The family and friends of the cardiac patient need your guidance and reassurance. It's your job to make them know someone cares about their loved one and his family.

Documenting your assessment

Patient name: _Arthur Dorn_

Age: _62_

Diagnosis: _CHF_

Room: _207_

Doctor: _Prynne_

Temp: _99° F_

Resp: _32 regular, shallow_

Pulse: _Radial 105 Apical 115_

B/P: _158/96_

Cardiac assessment form

Head-to-toe inspection:

Extremities: color: _pale_

temperature: _cool and moist_

clubbing: _none_

hair growth: _sparse on calves_

edema: _+3 pretibial +1 pedal_

Venous blood pressure: _distended jugular veins_

Arterial pulses:

	Rate	Rhythm	Arterial wall	Amplitude	Bilateral equality
carotid:	100	regular	rope-like	+2	yes
brachial:	100	regular	rope-like	+2	yes
radial:	100	regular	rope-like	+2	yes
femoral:	100	regular	rope-like	+2	yes
popliteal:	100	regular	rope-like	+2	yes
posterior tibial:	100	regular	rope-like	+1	yes
dorsalis pedis:	100	regular	rope-like	+1	yes

Breath sounds: _moist rales in bases bilaterally_

Heart examination:

Inspection: pulsations: _none_

Palpation: PMI: _5th ICS 3cm to left of midclavicular line_

thrills: _over aortic area_

heaves: _over left ventricular area_

pulsations: _over left ventricular area_

Percussion: heart border location _4cm 4th ICS, 10cm 5th ICS, 12cm 6th ICS_

Auscultation: S₁: _normal_

S₂: _no split on inspiration_

S₃: _present_

S₄: _present_

Murmurs: location: _aortic area URSB_

timing: _systolic, ejection_

radiation: _apex and carotid arteries_

loudness: _grade 4_

pitch: _high_

intensity: _crescendo-decrescendo_

quality: _harsh_

Signature of nurse: _Dorothy Jovinelly, RN_

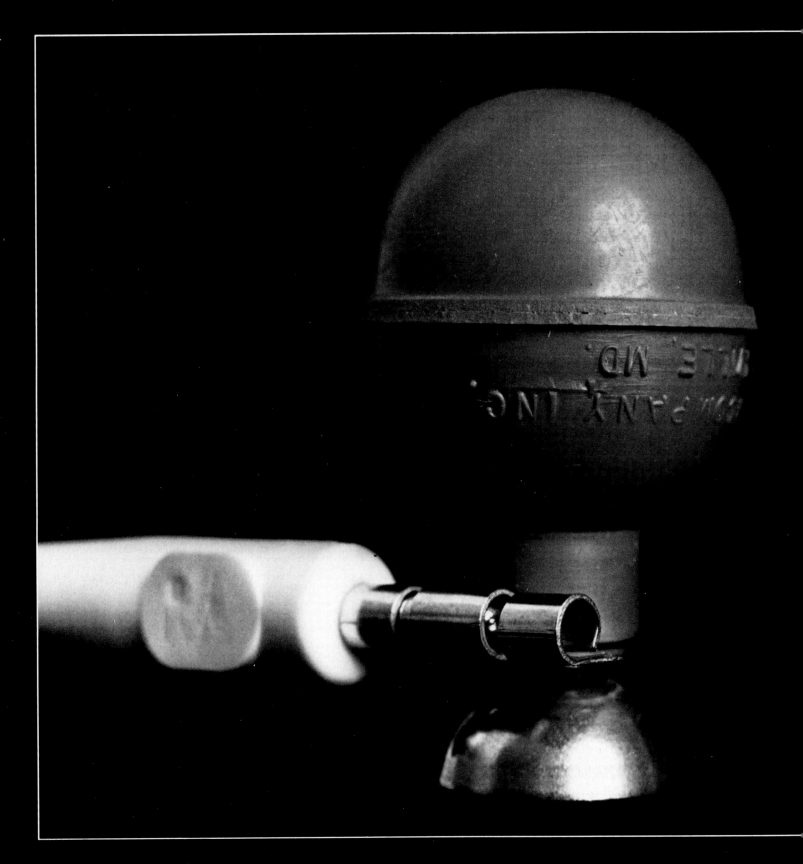

Performing Diagnostic Tests

Cardiography

Radiography

Sonic tests

Pulse wave tracings

Invasive tests

Cardiography

Ever run a 12-lead electro-cardiogram (EKG)? Don't be intimidated, because it really isn't difficult. By following the proper procedure carefully, you can produce highly diagnostic readout strips that'll help the doctor evaluate your patient's condition.

In the next few pages, you'll see exactly how to run a 12-lead EKG. In addition, you'll learn how to use the EKG to test artificial pacemaker function.

Suppose, despite your best efforts, you can't produce clear readout strips. To help you correct this problem, we've provided a special trouble-shooting chart. We've also included lots of background information on how EKGs work and how to interpret them, so you can answer your patient's questions accurately and completely.

What if your patient's scheduled for a vectorcar-diogram, a cardiogram that represents the heart's electrical activity in three dimensions? Although you won't do the procedure yourself, you're responsible for teaching your patient about it. In this chapter, you'll also learn how to prepare him for vectorcar-diography.

Understanding the 12-lead EKG

If you've ever cared for a patient recovering from a myocardial infarction, you're familiar with electrocardiograms (EKGs). But most likely, you're not quite sure how and why the EKG works.

No wonder. It's a complicated subject. But the information on this page will give you enough background to understand the basics of the standard 12-lead EKG.

As you know, the cardiac cycle depends on electrical processes within the heart: depolarization and repolarization. Following depolarization, the myocardium contracts; following repolarization, it relaxes. (For a review of electrical conduction during the cardiac cycle, see page 38.)

During depolarization and repolarization, charged ions move back and forth across myocardial cell membranes. This movement creates a flow of electrical current that radiates in all directions from the heart. The force of this current is called *electrical potential*. Electrodes placed on the skin measure electrical potential as the current reaches the skin's surface.

Keep in mind that an EKG can measure only *electrical* energy. It can't directly measure mechanical events, like myocardial contractions. However, by studying the electrical patterns on an EKG strip, you can draw valuable conclusions about myocardial function.

A 12-lead EKG examines the heart's electrical potential from 12 different views. As a result, it gives a more complete picture of the heart than hardwire, or continuous, monitoring.

Each of these 12 views is called a *lead*. The 12 leads are the standard limb leads (I, II, III), the augmented limb leads (AVR, AVL, AVF), and the chest, or precordial, leads (V_1 through V_6).

Now, let's take a closer look at the standard limb leads: I, II, and III. To run these three leads, you'll place a limb electrode on each of the patient's arms and legs—four electrodes in all. (You'll see exactly how to do this in the photostory on pages 41 to 45.) Because the electrode on your patient's right leg acts as the ground, it's inactive.

The EKG machine compares electrical potential flowing between two of the three active electrodes. These three leads are called *bipolar* leads. When active, the right arm electrode is always the negative pole and the left leg electrode is always the positive pole. But the left arm electrode's charge is changeable. For lead I, it's positive; for lead III, it's negative. (The left arm electrode is inactive for lead II.) The EKG machine will read the direction of electrical potential according to how you set the machine's lead selector.

Now, let's look at the augmented limb leads: AVR, AVL, and AVF. In these abbreviations, the A means augmented; V means voltage; and R, L, and F mean right arm, left arm, and foot, respectively. These three leads use the same electrode placement as standard limb leads.

Unlike the standard limb leads, however, the augmented limb leads are *unipolar*. What's the difference? Instead of measuring electrical potential between a positive and a negative electrode, the EKG machine measures electrical potential between one limb lead electrode and the electrical midpoint between the remaining two electrodes. The EKG machine determines this midpoint electronically.

But the standard and augmented limb leads are alike in this respect: they both measure electrical potential in the body's *frontal* plane (see the illustration on the next page). In other words, they view your patient's heart from the front.

Now, let's discuss the six chest (precordial) leads: V_1 through V_6. To run these leads, you'll place a fifth electrode on your patient's chest. The numbers indicate the position of the electrode on the chest wall. You'll place the chest electrode in a different position for each of the six chest leads (see the illustration on page 40).

The chest leads also are unipolar. To run a chest lead, the EKG machine averages the electrical potentials of all three active limb lead electrodes. Then, it electronically compares this average with the electrical potential of the chest electrode.

As the illustration on the next page shows, the chest leads add still another dimension to the EKG picture. Whereas the standard and augmented limb leads view electrical potential from the body's frontal plane, the chest leads view the electrical potential from a horizontal plane. This added dimension helps pinpoint any damage to the heart's lateral or posterior walls.

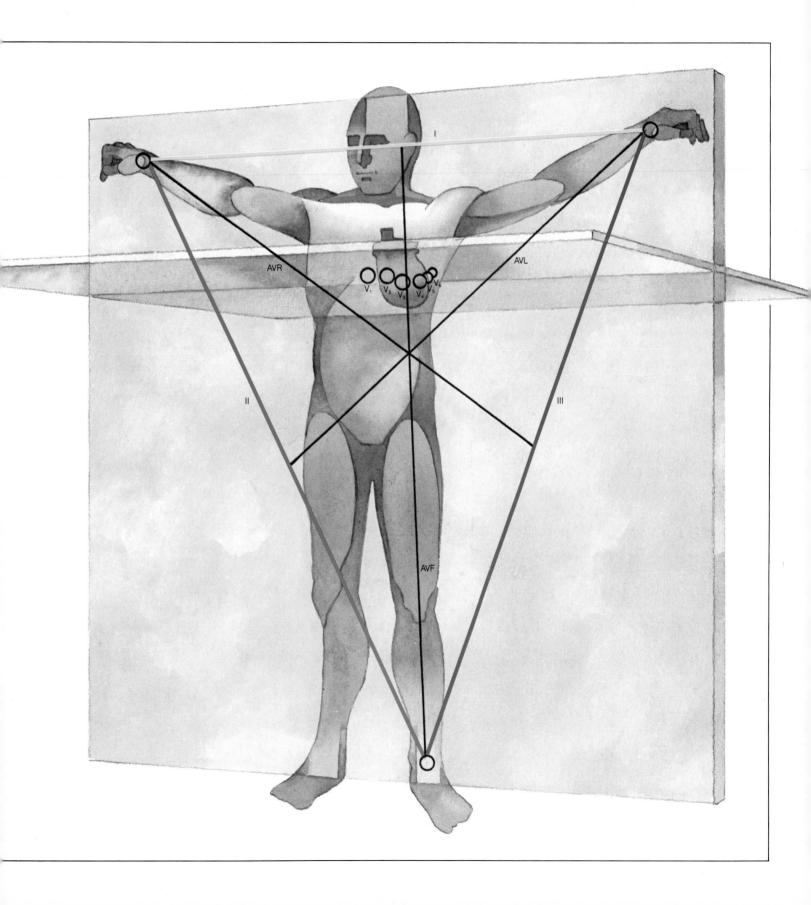

Cardiography

EKG waveforms: What they tell us

You're already familiar with the EKG. As you know, it reflects electrical activity in the heart. But can you interpret each deflection of the EKG waveform? If not, look at the illustration below. The corresponding colors show how the EKG waveform reflects cardiac conduction.

Electrical stimulation of the heart originates in the sinoatrial (SA) node, which is the heart's sparkplug, or pacemaker. As you can see in the illustration below, the SA node is located in the upper wall of the right atrium. With regularity, it sends electrical impulses to the atria, stimulating them to contract. The P wave on the EKG waveform appears as the atria depolarize.

Next, the electrical impulse travels to the atrioventricular (AV) junction, where it's slowed. This slowing-down process allows the heart's ventricles to fill with blood from the atria. As this happens, the waveform briefly returns to baseline for the P-R interval. A normal P-R interval lasts approximately 0.12 to 0.2 seconds, and indicates the amount of time it takes an electrical impulse to travel from the SA node through the atria and the atrioventricular junction into the ventricles.

From the AV junction, the impulse travels down the bundle of His, the left and right bundle branches, and the Purkinje fibers.

As the impulse stimulates the ventricles, they contract and eject blood into the pulmonary artery and the aorta. As cells in the ventricles depolarize, the QRS complex appears. Then, the EKG waveform briefly returns to baseline in the S-T segment.

As you can see in the illustration, the Q wave is a negative (downward) deflection; the R wave's a positive (upward) deflection; and the S wave's a negative deflection that follows the R wave. A QRS interval lasts approximately 0.06 to 0.1 seconds. *Note:* Some leads don't display all three waves of the QRS complex.

Finally, the cells in the ventricles repolarize, producing a T wave. Occasionally, the T wave's followed by a U wave, indicating repolarization of Purkinje fiber cells. You'll see prominent or inverted U waves if your patient has bradycardia, hypokalemia, or ventricular hypertrophy.

Note: If electrical impulses from the SA node are suppressed or blocked, the AV junction usually takes over and maintains a heart rate of 40 to 60 beats per minute. If the AV junction's impulses are also blocked, ventricular cells initiate electrical conduction. However, the ventricular cells can maintain a heart rate of only 20 to 40 beats per minute.

Preparing your patient for a 12-lead EKG

Millie Harvey, a 52-year-old telephone operator, watches you roll a cold, gray EKG machine to her bedside. She knows her doctor has scheduled her for an EKG (although she isn't quite sure what an EKG is), and she figures the machine has something to do with it. Apprehensively, she asks, "Will it hurt?" What do you say?

Immediately assure her that the procedure won't hurt—in fact, she won't feel a thing. But don't stop there. Explain how the EKG works and how it can help you and the doctor correctly treat her condition. Then, if she's alert and comfortable, make your explanation of the EKG clearer by reviewing some basics about her heart and how it works. Whenever possible, *show* her EKG strips and illustrations, such as the one to the left, to increase her understanding.

Use terms she knows. Don't use a complicated word or a medical term if a simple, everyday one is just as accurate. For instance, why confuse your patient with a term such as *ectopy*, when *irregular heartbeat* will serve as well?

Don't skip this important part of patient preparation, even if your patient's had an EKG before. Maybe no one's ever explained the procedure before. Or, perhaps she was too sick or anxious to understand what she was told. Find out how much she's learned; then, supplement her knowledge, if necessary.

The dialogue on the following page suggests some common questions and misconceptions patients like Mrs. Harvey have. Use it as a guide when you teach. Then, encourage your patient to ask her own questions. This'll give you the chance to clear up remaining misunderstandings.

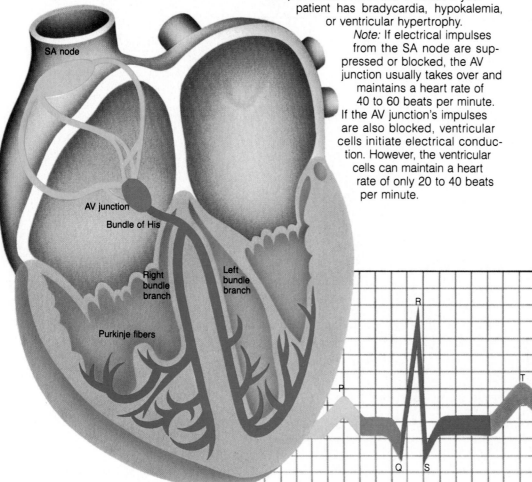

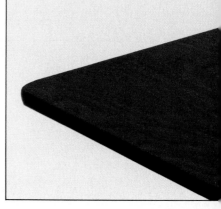

Patient's question: What *is* an EKG, anyway?

Your answer: The term EKG—or sometimes ECG—is an abbreviation for electrocardiogram. When interpreted by a trained person, the EKG shows your heart's electrical activity.

Patient's question: My heart's electrical activity? I thought the heart works like a pump.

Your answer: It does, but think of it as a pump with its own built-in power generator, which in the heart is called the *sinus node*. The sinus node—or SA node—is a specialized group of cells located in the upper right portion of the heart. Each second (approximately), it releases an electrical current that travels down a pathway of special muscle fibers—the heart's electrical wiring—and spreads throughout the heart. This current stimulates the heart muscle to contract and pump blood through the heart's chambers and finally into your body's vascular system. Then, the current spreads throughout your whole body, even reaching the skin on your fingers and toes, although you can't feel it.

Patient's question: How does the EKG work?

Your answer: With the help of five electrodes I'll put on your arms, legs, and chest, the EKG machine will record, on paper, these electrical currents as they reach your skin. Once recorded, these currents are called EKG waveforms. The strip of paper that comes out of the machine is called an *EKG waveform strip*.

Patient's question: What are electrodes?

Your answer: Electrodes are conductors that pick up your heart's electrical signals as they reach your skin. For your EKG, I'll apply two different types. The electrodes I'll put on your arms and legs are small metal rectangles, which are held in place with rubber straps. But the electrode I'll put on your chest is held in place by suction, so it has a rubber bulb on top of it. I'll place a special jelly under each electrode to help it pick up your heart's electrical signals clearly. This jelly may feel cold.

Patient's question: You'll apply five different electrodes. Why do I need so many?

Your answer: The four electrodes on your arms and legs view your heart's electrical signals from six different directions. The chest electrode, which I'll reposition several times during the procedure, allows us to view the heart from six more directions, for a total of 12 views. By examining the heart from these 12 different directions, the EKG test gives a nearly complete picture of the heart's electrical activity.

Patient's question: What does the EKG machine tell the doctor about my heart?

Your answer: By studying the EKG strips, the doctor can detect possible disturbances in your heart's electrical system. Since he knows which view each portion of the strip represents, he can locate damaged heart muscle that interrupts or blocks normal electrical activity.

Patient's question: Will one EKG be enough?

Your answer: No, the doctor will probably want you to have additional EKGs as you recover. By studying the EKG strips, your doctor can judge how quickly and completely your heart's healing.

Patient's question: Can the EKG machine give me a shock?

Your answer: No, EKGs are safe and painless. EKG equipment only measures electrical activity already present in your body. It doesn't conduct any electricity into your body.

Patient's question: What do I do during the procedure?

Your answer: Just lie flat and relax. Breathe normally and keep your arms and legs still. And don't talk—talking may distort the recordings, and make them inaccurate.

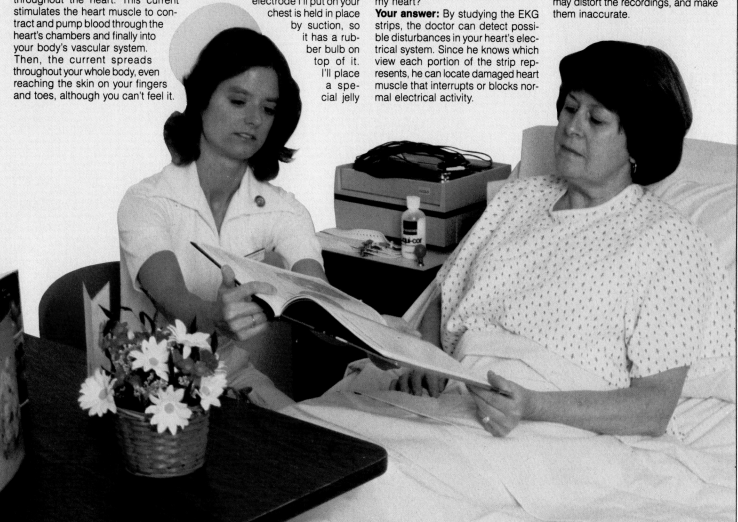

Cardiography

Marking an EKG strip

Planning to run a 12-lead EKG? As you work, you'll use the MARK button on the EKG machine to identify each lead. By pushing the button, you'll imprint a code of short and long dashes directly onto the EKG strip.

The code shown below is employed widely, although your EKG machine may use another one automatically. To avoid confusion, check the manufacturer's instructions.

Limb leads

I: −

II: − −

III: − − −

AVR: − ——

AVL: − − ——

AVF: − − − ——

Chest leads

V_1:   —— −

V_2:   —— − −

V_3:   —— − − −

V_4:   —— − − − −

V_5:   —— − − − − —

V_6:   —— − − − − − —

How to position chest electrodes correctly

You probably know that you must position the chest electrode in different spots for each of the six chest leads (leads V_1 through V_6) of a 12-lead EKG. But do you know *exactly* where each position is? If not, examine this illustration. Then, read the following photostory to learn how to take a 12-lead EKG.

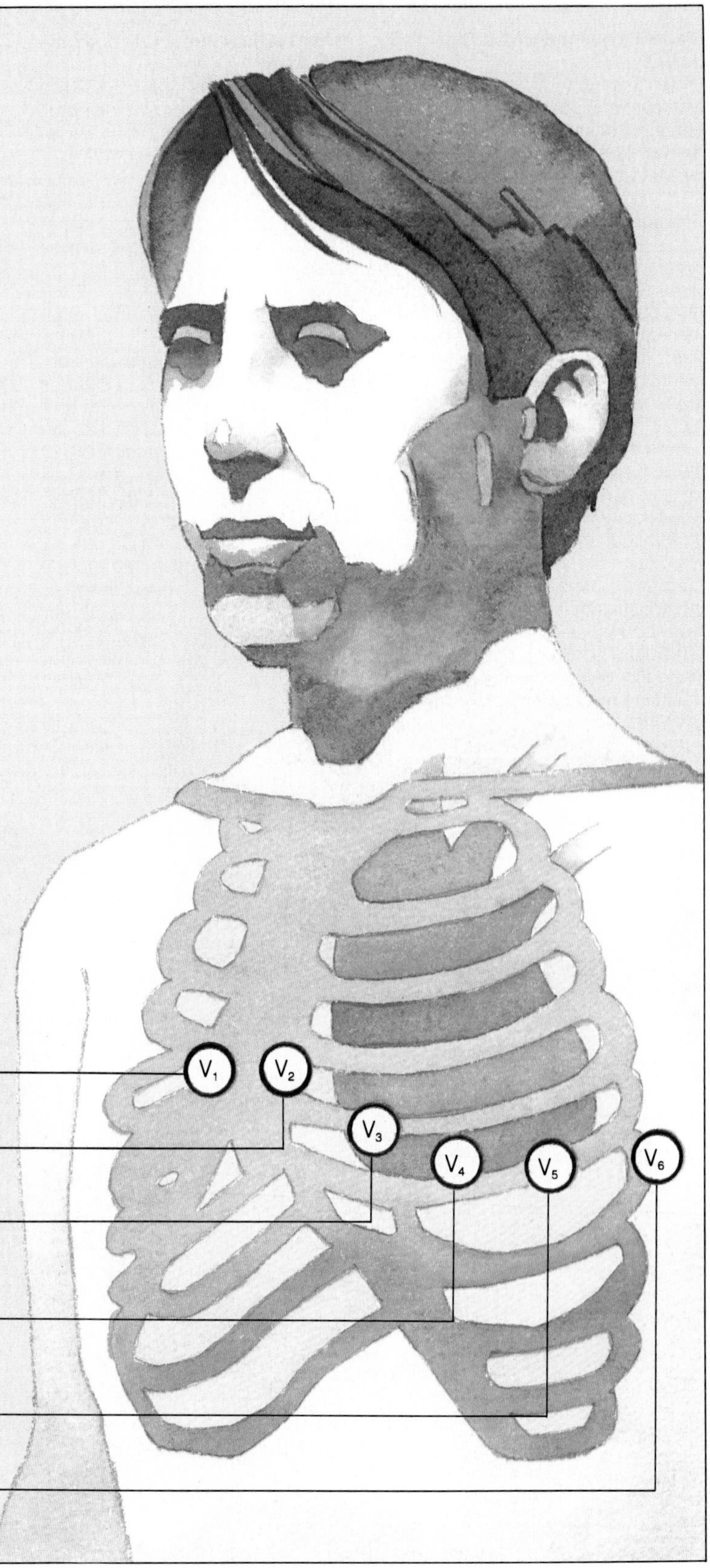

V_1: Fourth intercostal space to right of sternum

V_2: Fourth intercostal space to left of sternum

V_3: Halfway between V_2 and V_4

V_4: Fifth intercostal space at midclavicular line

V_5: Anterior axillary line (halfway between V_4 and V_6)

V_6: Midaxillary line, level with V_4

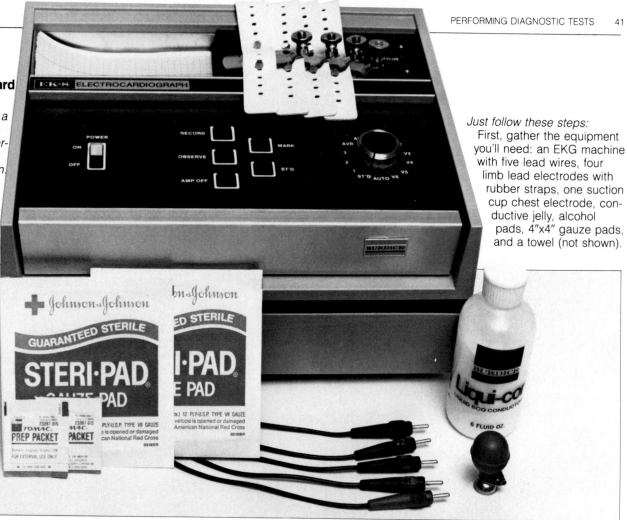

Running a standard 12-lead EKG

1 *William Hanson, a 55-year-old auto mechanic, is recovering from his second myocardial infarction. To help assess his progress, his doctor's ordered a 12-lead EKG. Can you do the procedure correctly?*

Just follow these steps: First, gather the equipment you'll need: an EKG machine with five lead wires, four limb lead electrodes with rubber straps, one suction cup chest electrode, conductive jelly, alcohol pads, 4"x4" gauze pads, and a towel (not shown).

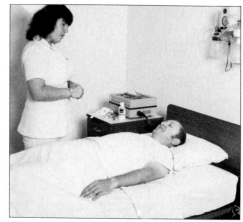

2 Place Mr. Hanson flat on his back, and make sure his feet don't touch the bed's footboard. Even though Mr. Hanson's had EKGs done before, discuss the procedure with him and answer his questions. (For guidelines on preparing a patient for an EKG, see pages 38 and 39.)

When you're sure Mr. Hanson understands the procedure, remove his gown and expose his arms and lower legs.
Note: Your patient may be embarrassed when you remove his gown. If he is, use a towel or sheet to cover him until you apply the chest electrode.

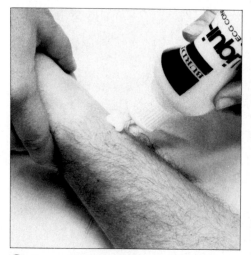

3 To apply limb lead electrodes to the patient's arms, first select a flat, fleshy site. Avoid bony or muscular areas. Then, place a small daub of conductive jelly on the site. As you see in this photo, the nurse has selected a site near the patient's wrist.

📠 *Nursing tip:* If conductive jelly isn't available, use a pad soaked with normal saline solution or alcohol. Either will conduct electrical impulses from the patient's skin to the electrode.

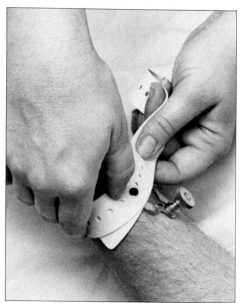

4 Place one of the limb lead electrodes on top of the jelly. Secure the electrode with a rubber strap, as shown here. *Note:* Avoid pulling the rubber strap too tight. Doing so may cause muscle spasms that'll distort the EKG readings.

Follow the same procedure to apply a limb lead electrode to the other wrist.

Cardiography

Running a standard 12-lead EKG continued

5 Then, choose a flat, fleshy site on one of the patient's legs and repeat the procedure. In this photo, the nurse has chosen a fleshy area near the ankle. Apply the fourth limb lead electrode to the patient's other leg, using the same procedure.

Nursing tip: Place the leg electrodes so their lead wire connectors point up the leg. This way, you can connect the lead wires to them without bending or straining the wires.

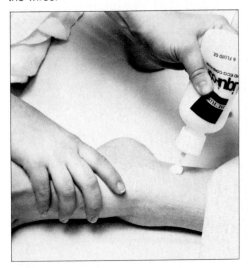

6 Next, match each limb lead electrode to the corresponding lead wire. Each lead wire is color coded as follows: white (right arm), black (left arm), green (right leg), red (left leg), and brown (chest). In addition, lead wires usually are coded with initials.

Connect each limb lead wire to the appropriate electrode. To do this, simply plug the lead wire prong into the electrode's lead wire connector. Secure it by turning the electrode screw, as shown here.

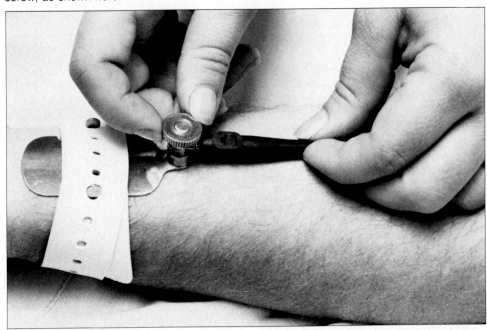

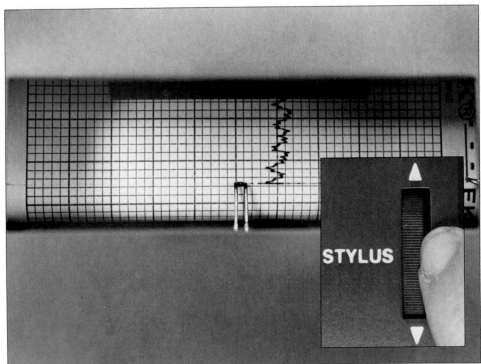

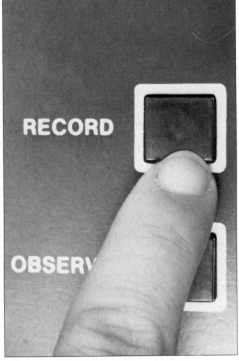

7 To turn on the EKG machine, depress the POWER switch. Then, make sure the stylus rests in the center of the EKG paper, as shown here. If it doesn't, adjust the STYLUS wheel, as shown in the inset photo.

8 If all's OK, press the RECORD button. The stylus will draw a straight baseline on the middle of the EKG paper.

9 To standardize (calibrate) the EKG machine, turn the lead selector to ST'D (standardize); then, press the ST'D button, as shown in the inset photo. As shown in the larger photo, you'll see a square wave that's 1 millivolt high (the height of 2 large squares on the EKG paper). To provide a consistent frame of reference throughout the procedure, standardize the machine after you run each lead. *Note:* The machine used here automatically standardizes itself. If the one you're using doesn't, the square wave may be more or less than 1 millivolt high. To learn how to standardize this type of machine, check the operator's manual.

10 Now you're ready to run the first six leads: I, II, III, AVR, AVL, and AVF. To begin, turn the lead selector knob to 1 (lead I) and run a 6-second strip.

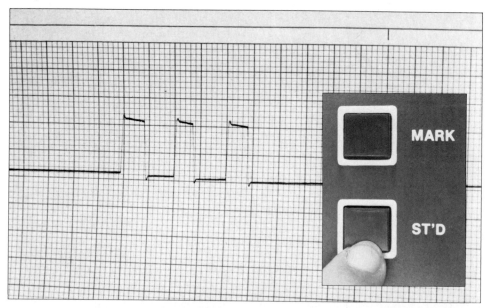
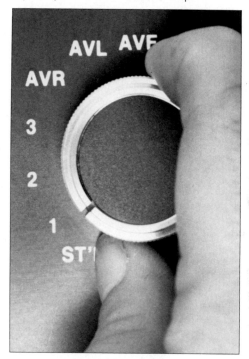

11 As the strip runs, press the MARK button to mark the strip with one short dash, the code for lead I. (For a review of EKG lead codes, see the chart on page 40.)

[Inset] Press the AMP OFF button to stop the strip. *Note:* If you prefer, you may stop the strip by pressing the OBSERVE button.

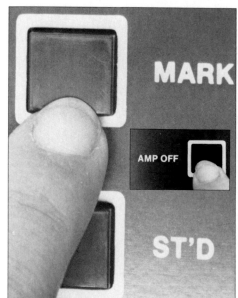

12 Then, turn the lead selector to 2 (lead II) and run another 6-second strip. Mark the strip with the correct code (two short dashes). Repeat this procedure until you've run and marked 6-second strips for leads III, AVR, AVL, and AVF. *Note:* If you observe ectopic beats or rhythm changes, run longer strips, so the doctor can observe these irregularities at greater length.

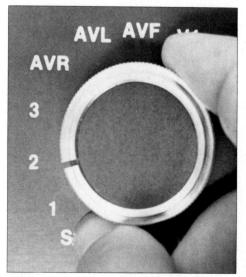

13 Now, you're ready to apply the chest electrode. Expose the patient's chest, if you haven't already, and place a daub of conductive jelly at the V, position (fourth intercostal space to the right of the patient's sternum). Pick up the chest electrode and squeeze its rubber bulb between your fingers. Place the electrode on the jelly and release the rubber bulb. Suction will hold the electrode in place.

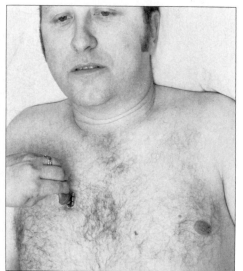

Cardiography

Running a standard 12-lead EKG continued

14 Attach the brown chest lead wire to the chest electrode, as the nurse is doing here.

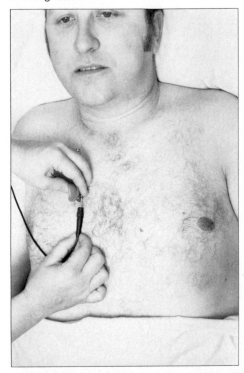

15 To run the first chest lead, set the lead selector on V_1, as shown here. Then, press the RECORD button and run a 6-second V_1 strip. As the strip runs, remember to mark it properly.

To stop the strip, press the AMP OFF button.

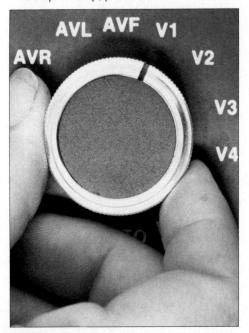

16 You must reposition the chest electrode to run each of the five remaining chest leads. To run lead V_2, move the chest electrode to V_2 position, as shown below. (If you're unsure about chest lead positions, review the illustration on page 40.) If the electrode won't adhere firmly, apply more conductive jelly.

Now, press the RECORD button. Run and mark a 6-second strip; then, stop the strip. Repeat this procedure to run strips for all the chest leads.

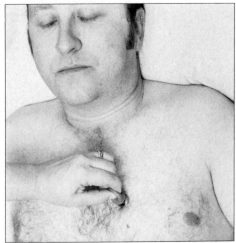

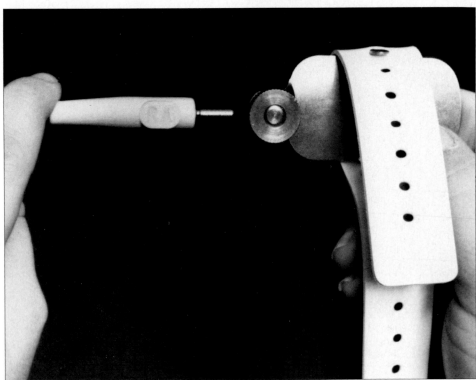

17 When the EKG's complete, remove the electrodes from the patient's skin. Then, disconnect the lead wires from the electrodes.

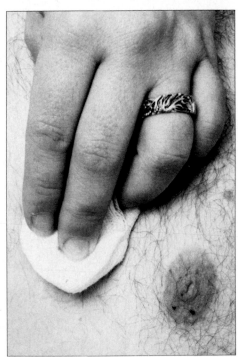

18 Use 4"x4" gauze pads to clean the conductive jelly from his skin, as shown here. Help him back into his gown or pajamas, and position him comfortably.

19 Using alcohol pads, clean the limb lead electrodes, as shown here. To clean the chest electrode, hold it under running water. Then, return them to their drawer.

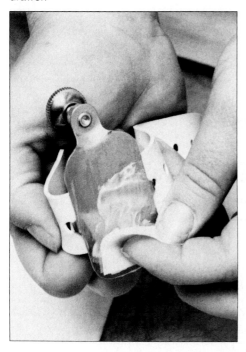

20 Document the entire procedure. On the back of each EKG strip, write the patient's name and room number, his age, the date and time of the procedure, the doctor's name, and your initials. In addition, include any other special information about your patient. For instance, does he have an artificial pacemaker? Did he feel any chest pain during the EKG? Was electrode placement unusual because he's an amputee, or wearing a cast? If so, write it down. Then, mount the EKG strip on his chart or send it to the EKG department, according to hospital policy.

> William Hanson
> Room 203
> 55 y/o
> 11/10/80
> 10 AM
> Dr. Rose
> L.G.

Dealing with special problems

Does your patient's physical condition or age present a problem when he needs an EKG? Here's how to deal with some special situations:

Patient is an amputee
• Place the limb lead electrode on his stump.
• If no stump remains, place the limb lead electrode on the trunk near the amputation site.
• Document the unusual electrode placement, and the reason for it.

Patient has severe burns
• Use sterile electrodes.
• Clean the EKG machine carefully before the procedure to minimize the risk of infection.
• If the patient's in reverse isolation, follow the hospital's infection control policy.

Patient has a limb cast
• You may place the electrode under the cast, but make sure it lies flat against his skin.
• Or, place the electrode on skin above cast.
• Document the unusual electrode placement, and the reason for it.

Patient has dextrocardia (heart on right side of chest)
• Run a regular 12-lead EKG. Then, reverse the arm leads and run leads V_2 through V_6 on the right side of his chest. Mark the additional strips like this: $V_2(R)$, $V_3(R)$, $V_4(R)$, $V_5(R)$, $V_6(R)$. In addition, note that you reversed the arm leads.
• Document the unusual procedure, and the reason for it.

Patient is an infant or child (under age 14)
• Use smaller electrodes, proportional to the child's size.
• Run a regular 12-lead EKG. Then, run leads V_3 and V_4 on the right side of his chest, because a child's heart lies less to the left than an adult's. Mark the additional strips like this: $V_3(R)$ and $V_4(R)$.
• Document the unusual procedure, and the reason for it.

> William Hanson
> Room 203
>
> DATE 11/10/80
>
> **ELECTROCARDIOGRAM**
>
> □ O.P. REF.   □ E.D.   □ P.A.T.
>
> □ O.P. CLINIC   □ I.P.   □ OTHER
>
> REQUESTED BY   CHARGE NURSE
> Dr. Rose   L. Gilge
>
> **REQUEST**
>
> DIAGNOSIS Anterior MI
>
> CIRCLE MEDICATIONS IN USE—(DIGITALIS)—KCL—PRONESTYL—QUINIDINE
>
> DIURETIC—(INDERAL)—DILANTIN—ATROPINE—OTHERS
>
> BLOOD PRESSURE 104/74   PULSE 104   RESPIRATORY 22
>
> WEIGHT 190   HEIGHT 5'8"   AGE 55   SEX M

21 If you send the strip to the EKG department, fill out the EKG request form completely. Include this information: the patient's age, height, weight, blood pressure, and diagnosis. Also, include the name of any medication he's taking, as well as other special information.

Cardiography

Recognizing EKG waveforms

When you run a 12-lead EKG, you'll notice that each lead's waveform is distinctive. The reason, of course, is that each lead reflects the heart's electrical activity from a different view.

These illustrations show typical waveforms for each of the 12 leads. Notice that leads AVR, V_1, V_2, and V_3 show strong negative deflections; that is, deflections *below* the baseline. This is normal for those leads. Negative deflections simply show that the electrical current's flowing away from the positive electrode. Likewise, positive deflections (deflections *above* the baseline) show that the electrical current's flowing toward the positive electrode.

Take special note of the lead II waveform. Because it most clearly depicts the heart's rhythm, it's sometimes called the *rhythm strip*.

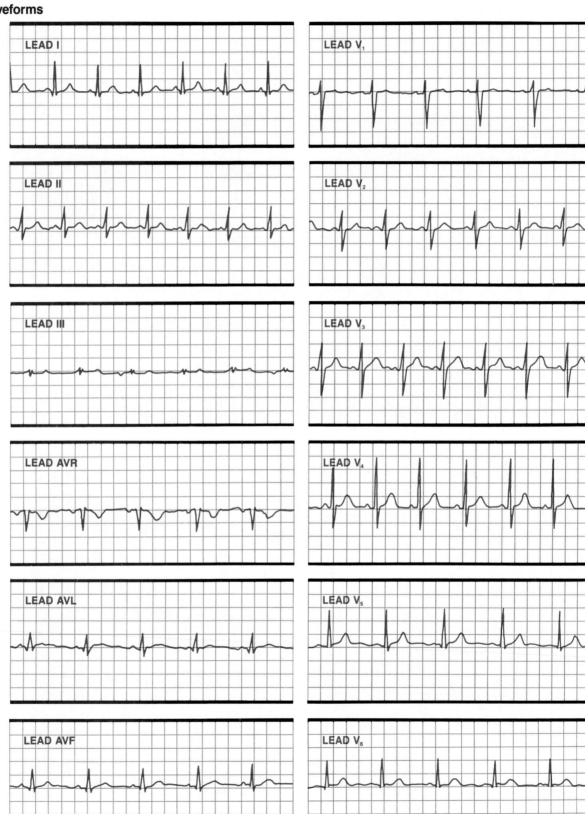

Interpreting an EKG

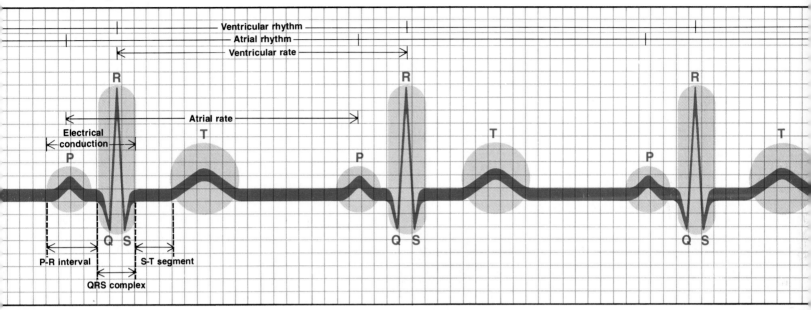

To read an EKG correctly, you must first examine the waveform to gather some basic information from it. Do you know what this basic information is? Read what follows:

• *Heart rhythm:* You can determine whether or not your patient's heart rhythm is regular or irregular by measuring the distance between each wave in a series. To determine atrial rhythm, measure the distance between two P waves, using calipers or a piece of paper. Tighten the calipers, or mark the piece of paper to indicate this distance. Then, using this marked-off distance, compare it with the distances between other P waves on the EKG strip. If the distance between each wave is exactly the same, your patient's atrial rhythm is regular. If the distance varies slightly, his atrial rhythm's slightly irregular. If it varies markedly, his atrial rhythm is considered markedly irregular.

To determine your patient's ventricular rhythm, repeat the entire measuring procedure, using the QRS complexes. Measure from R wave to R wave.

• *Heart rate:* As you probably know, you're measuring only your patient's ventricular heart rate when you take his pulse. But you can measure both his ventricular and atrial heart rates from his EKG.

If your patient's heart rhythm is *regular,* follow these steps:

Since the P wave represents atrial activity, you'll use this wave to determine your patient's atrial heart rate. Study two consecutive P waves. Select identical points on each; for example, the waves' starting points or their apex. Then, count the number of squares between these two points.

Each square represents 0.04 seconds. That means that 1,500 squares equal 1 minute. Since you want to find the atrial heart rate per minute, divide 1,500 by the number of squares you counted between P waves. The quotient is your patient's atrial heart rate.

Now, repeat the procedure with the QRS complex, measuring from R to R. This will tell you your patient's ventricular heart rate.

If your patient's heart rhythm is *irregular,* follow this procedure instead:

To determine the atrial heart rate, count the number of P waves within the space of 30 large blocks. Since each small block is equal to 0.04 seconds, and it takes five small blocks to make up one large block, each large block equals 0.2 seconds. Thirty large blocks, therefore, equal 6 seconds. Take the number of P waves you counted within 30 large blocks (6 seconds), and multiply it by 10 to get your patient's atrial rate for 1 minute.

To determine ventricular rate for the patient with an irregular rhythm, repeat the same calculations, this time counting QRS complexes instead.

• *Electrical conduction.* Conduction refers to the time it takes for an electrical impulse originating in the heart's SA node to stimulate ventricular contraction. To determine conduction time, measure the P-R interval and the duration of the QRS complex.

To measure the P-R interval, count the squares between the beginning of the P wave and the beginning of the R wave. Then, multiply this number by 0.04 seconds. The product represents how long it took an electrical impulse to travel from the heart's SA node through the atrium to the ventricles. The normal time is 0.12 to 0.2 seconds.

Follow the same steps to find the duration of the QRS complex. Count the squares between the beginning of the Q wave and the end of the S wave. Multiply this number by 0.04 seconds to find out how long it took an electrical impulse to pass through the heart's ventricles. The normal time is 0.04 to 0.12 seconds.

• *Configuration and location.* Ask yourself these basic questions to determine the configuration and location of the wave pattern:

Are all the P waves the same size and shape? Do they point in the same direction? Do they precede QRS complexes? Are they all the same distance from the T waves that precede them?

Are all the QRS complexes the same shape and size? Do they point in the same direction? Do they precede T waves? Are they all the same distance from the T waves that follow them?

Are the S-T segments above or below the baseline? Do they line up with the P-R intervals?

Are all the T waves the same shape and size? Do they all point in the same direction? Do they all point in the same direction as the QRS complexes?

Knowing how to gather this basic information will help you learn how to read an EKG. Armed with this information, you can proceed to the chart on pages 152 and 153. In it, you'll learn what your observations tell about the electrical activity of your patient's heart.

Cardiography

Testing pacemaker function

1 *Consider this possibility: your patient has a permanently implanted demand pacemaker set at 75 beats per minute. As you know, a demand pacemaker fires only when the patient's heart rate drops below the preset rate. If the patient's heart rate exceeds the pacemaker's set rate, how can you be sure the pacemaker's reliable?*

If the doctor orders, you can run a simple test with an EKG machine that immediately tells you whether the pacemaker's working properly. You may perform this test separately or as part of a 12-lead EKG. Suppose you're doing the test as part of a 12-lead EKG. Here's what to do:

Gather the usual equipment needed for a 12-lead EKG (see page 41). The only other equipment you'll need is a magnet, like the one in this photo.

Note: Some pacemakers require magnets made specifically for them. Check your patient's pacemaker ID card for more information.

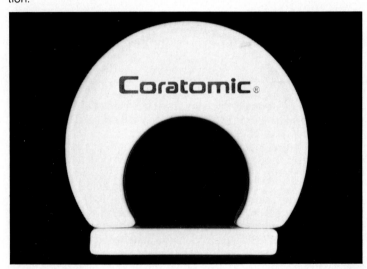

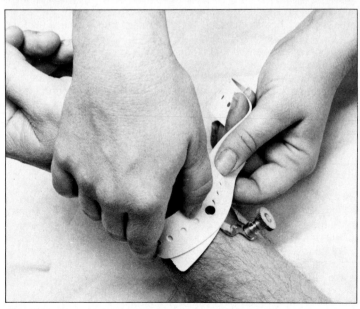

2 Place the electrodes and adjust the EKG machine as you usually would. Run and mark strips for lead I and lead II.

3 Leave the EKG machine's lead selector set for lead II. Then, hold the magnet about 1 inch (2.5 cm) directly above the pacemaker site, as the nurse is doing here. (Some magnets may be placed directly on the skin.) If the pacemaker's functioning properly, the magnet will cause it to fire regularly at a rate of 75 beats per minute.

Note: For some pacemakers, the magnet rate is faster than the set rate. This is normal for these pacemakers. Check the patient's pacemaker ID card.

Run a strip for about 1 minute. Then, set aside the magnet, and continue to run the other 10 leads, following the usual procedure.

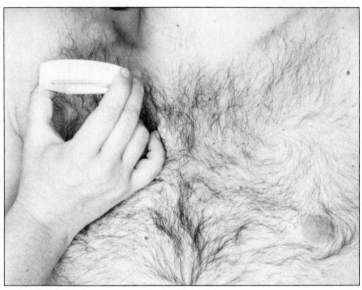

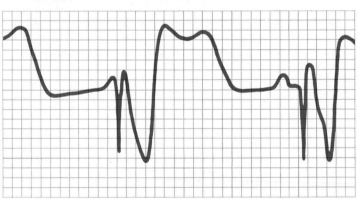

4 The lead II waveform illustrated above shows a regular 75 beat per minute rate. (Notice the spike preceding the QRS complex. This indicates that the pacemaker has fired.) But suppose your patient's unassisted heart rate is significantly higher than the pacemaker's set rate. Then your waveform will look less regular than the one shown here. Since the patient's heart continues to beat independently of the pacemaker, it creates a *competing rhythm*. As a result, a spike may not precede every QRS complex, and a QRS complex may not follow every spike.

Determine the pacemaker rate by calculating the distance between each spike, *not* each QRS complex. If the pacemaker didn't maintain a regular 75 beat per minute heart rate, notify the doctor.

Indicate on the strip that you used a magnet when you ran it. For more information, see the section on cardiac pacemakers.

Troubleshooting 12-lead EKGs

Suppose you see an unusual waveform on the 12-lead EKG strip you're running; a waveform like one of those shown below. What's the problem? And what should you do about it?

As always, make the patient your first concern. Check him imme- diately to see if the EKG reflects a change in his condition. But if you've ruled out this possibility, look for other causes. Use this chart as a guide.

Waveform	Possible cause	Solution
Jagged tracing, or thickened, fuzzy baseline	• Electrical interference (60-cycle interference) • Improper application of electrodes • Cracked or broken lead wires • Improper grounding of EKG machine	• Unplug other electrical equipment in the room, such as electric beds, heating pads, humidifiers, suction machines, and I.V. infusion pumps. • Reposition the electrodes on firm, fleshy areas of the patient's skin. Avoid bony prominences. • For better conduction between skin and electrode, replace alcohol or saline pads with conductive jelly. • Check for cracked or broken lead wires. Replace them, if necessary. • If your EKG machine has a separate ground wire, make sure it's clamped to a metal surface, such as a faucet.
Irregular, random deflections (artifact, or waveform interference)	• Patient movement, including talking and muscle tremors • Static electricity interference from nylon clothing or decrease in room humidity • Electrical short circuit in lead wires or cable • Improper application of electrodes • Poor connection between electrode and lead wire	• Encourage patient to relax. Wait until he's quiet to continue procedure. • Dress the patient in cotton, not nylon. Regulate room humidity to 40%. • Replace broken equipment. • Check electrodes and reposition them, if necessary. • Tighten electrode screw holding lead wire.
Wavy baseline	• Interference from an I.V. infusion pump • Patient movement • Atrial fibrillation	• Unplug pump during EKG. • Encourage patient to relax. • If baseline remains wavy, and you can't identify P waves, document atrial fibrillation pattern in your nurse's notes.
Wandering baseline; random, narrow deflections	• Muscle movement artifact • Improper application of electrodes	• Encourage patient to relax. Wait until he's quiet to continue procedure. • Check the rubber straps holding the limb electrodes in place, and loosen them, if necessary. Tight straps may cause muscle tremors. • Reposition electrodes on firm, fleshy sites. Avoid muscles and bony prominences. If the patient's elderly or thin, move the arm electrodes to fleshy sites on his upper arm.
Straight baseline	• Asystole • Improper connection of lead wire to electrode • Lead selector improperly set between leads, or on STD	• Check patient's condition. If he's asystolic, call a code and begin CPR. • Check cable and electrode connections and adjust them, if necessary. • Reposition lead selector.

Cardiography

Vectorcardiography: Learning the basics

Remember Millie Harvey? She's the patient you prepared for an EKG on pages 38 and 39. Now her EKG test results are back, and they suggest that she has a bundle branch block. But because the heart muscle surrounding the bundle branch was damaged during her myocardial infarction, Mrs. Harvey's EKG is too confusing to be conclusive. To clarify the EKG, the doctor orders a vectorcardiogram (VCG). By studying the VCG, he may be able to distinguish the heart's damaged areas.

Because you prepared Mrs. Harvey so well for her EKG, preparing her for a VCG is easy. Explain that the VCG is similar to the EKG, except that it views the heart's electrical activity from additional directions. As a result, it gives the doctor an even better picture of her heart's condition.

Assure Mrs. Harvey that the procedure's safe and painless. In fact, except for electrode placement, it's very much like an EKG. Tell her that a technician or nurse may place electrodes on her neck or forehead, in addition to her chest. (Electrode placement depends on the lead system the doctor chooses.)

Suppose Mrs. Harvey has questions. Can you answer them adequately? If you're not sure how VCGs work, you probably can't. The following information will improve your knowledge of VCG basics. With better understanding of this complex subject, you can answer Mrs. Harvey's questions confidently.

Comparing VCGs and EKGs

Like the EKG, the VCG records the heart's electrical activity through electrodes placed on the patient's skin. But a VCG differs from an EKG in one important way. An EKG provides a *two-dimensional* view of the heart along one of two planes, either horizontal or frontal. The VCG, on the other hand, views the heart from two of three planes. These planes are the horizontal plane, the frontal plane, and the left sagittal (or lateral) plane. By viewing the heart from two of these planes *simultaneously*, the VCG provides a *three-dimensional* picture of the heart.

That's why a VCG helps the doctor interpret a confusing EKG like Mrs. Harvey's, which suggested both a bundle branch block and myocardial damage. In addition, it may help the doctor to:
• identify atrial or ventricular enlargements that don't appear on the EKG.
• distinguish between some types of conduction disorders.

Measuring vectors

To understand VCGs fully, you must first understand vectors. Simply stated, vectors are composites of electrical potential from specific areas of the heart. Vectors have direction, magnitude, and polarity.

Vectors are measured along three axes, which correspond to three specific EKG leads. The horizontal axis (called X) corresponds to lead I; the vertical axis (called Y) corresponds to lead AVF; and the sagittal axis (called Z) corresponds to lead V_2.

The VCG combines two of these axes to form each plane:
• Combining axes X and Y produces the frontal plane.
• Combining axes X and Z produces the horizontal plane.
• Combining axes Z and Y produces the sagittal plane.

By viewing the heart from two of these planes at once, the VCG machine displays *vector loops*—loop-shaped, three-dimensional representations of the heart's electrical activity—on its oscilloscope screen. (The third plane is a reference point that checks the accuracy of the other two views.) To see how vector loops represent these planes, examine the illustration to the right.

Reading vector loops

Reading vector loops isn't easy: even the experts haven't agreed on standards for normal and abnormal loops. But the illustrations along the bottom of these pages will acquaint you with some of the basics.

As you see, a vector loop represents, with a series of dashes, the electrical activity of each heartbeat. The dashes end in an arrow, which represents the major thrust of electrical activity; in other words, the vector itself.

Each vector loop represents one complete cardiac cycle. As the illustrations show, segments of the vector loop correspond to the P, QRS, and T segments of an EKG waveform. By studying the shape of the loops, the spacing of the dashes, and the direction of the arrows, a doctor can detect abnormalities in the heart's electrical activity.

How VCGs correspond to EKGs

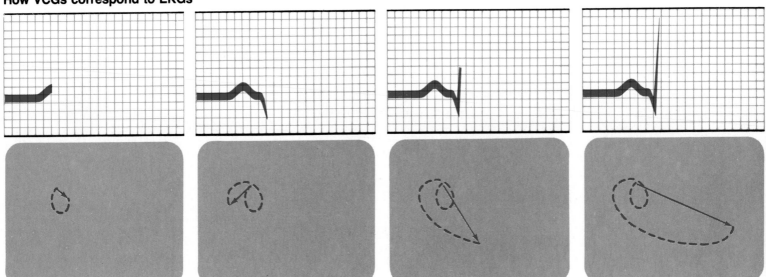

Cardiac conduction: A 3-dimensional view

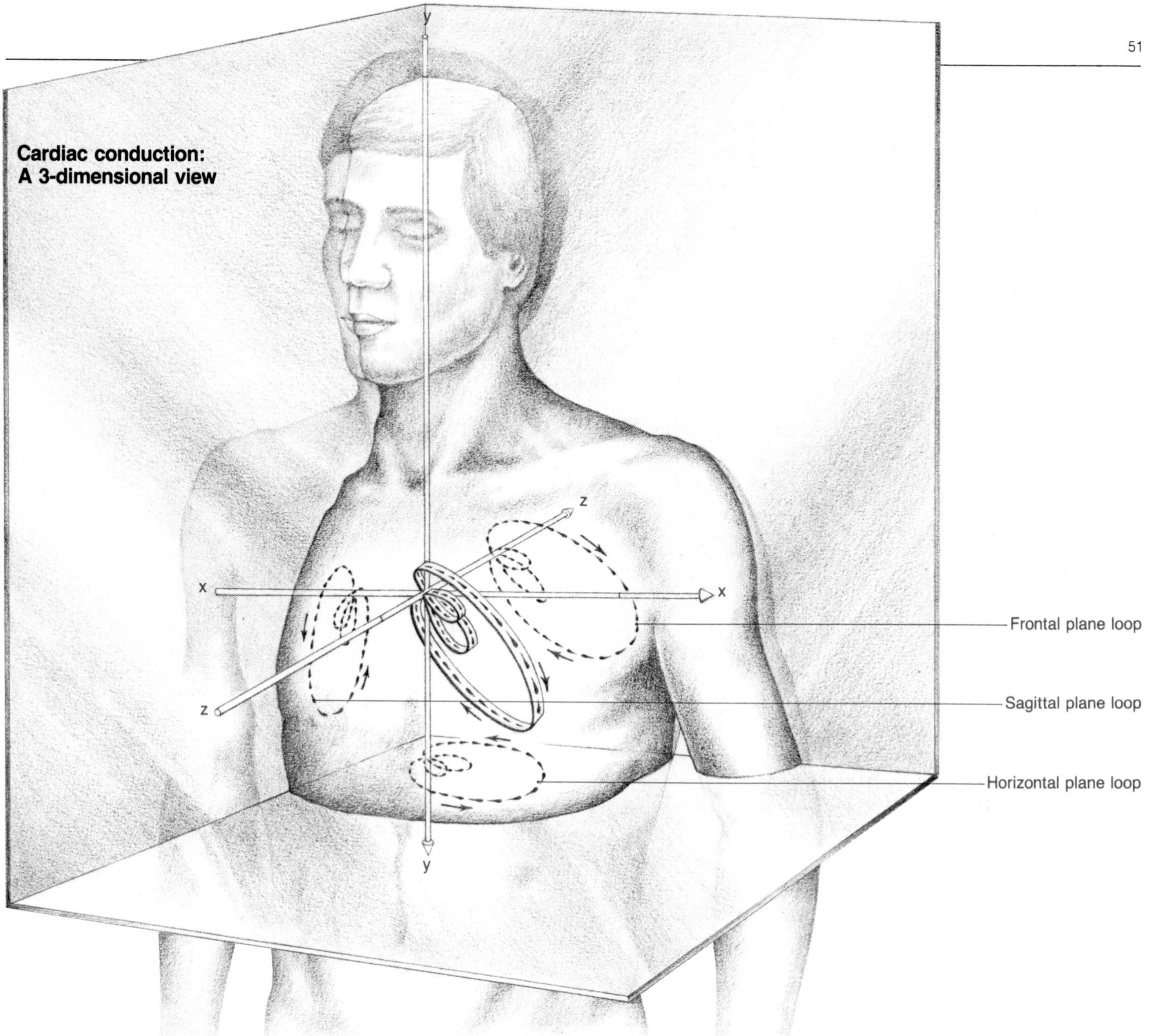
y
z
x
x
z
y
Frontal plane loop
Sagittal plane loop
Horizontal plane loop

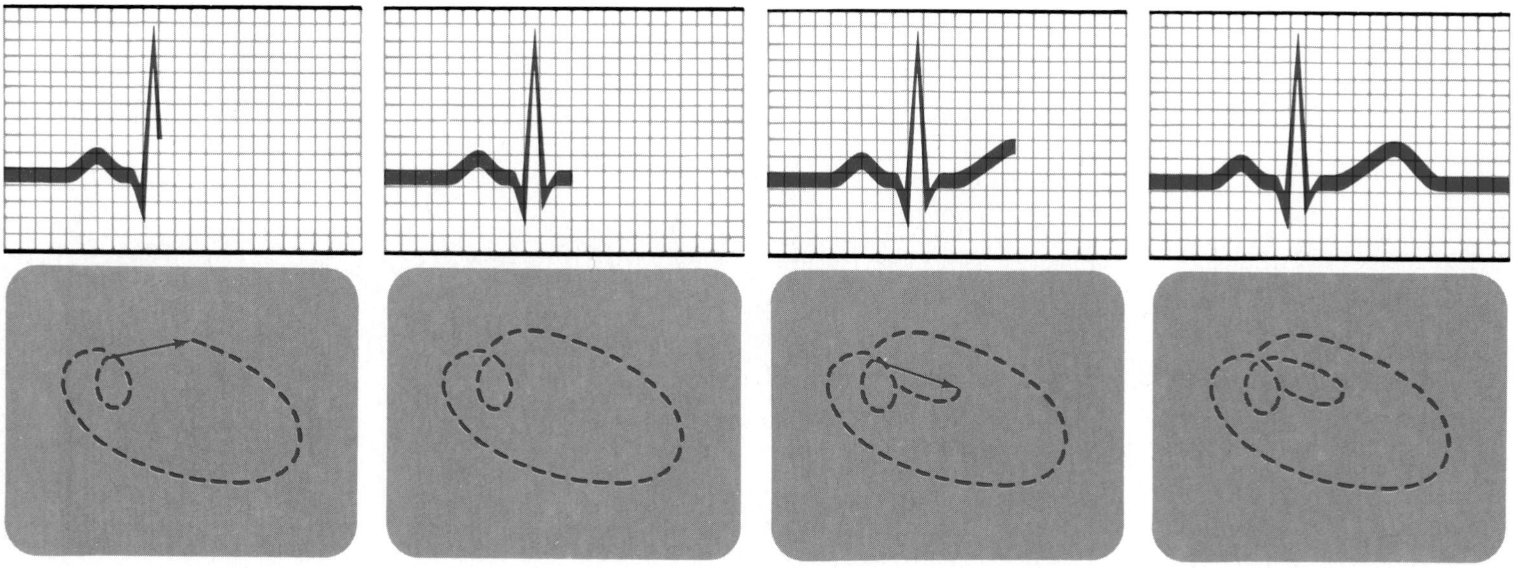

Radiography

Unlike the EKG, which records only electrical activity, radiography lets you look at the heart itself. The chest X-ray, perhaps the most common example of radiography, is nearly indispensable for evaluating heart disease. As a bonus, it also detects pulmonary congestion, which, in many cases, accompanies heart disease. Among the conditions radiography can help identify are:
• cardiac chamber enlargement
• cardiac calcifications
• pulmonary congestion caused by left-sided heart failure
• primary respiratory disease.

Fluoroscopy also visualizes the heart with X-rays. A closely related procedure, hot-spot imaging, visualizes the heart with gamma rays. In the following pages, you'll learn about all of these radiographic procedures. More important, you'll learn how to prepare your patient for them, and how to help him understand the results. With a solid background in radiography, you'll care for your patient completely and confidently.

PATIENT PREPARATION

Getting your patient ready for a chest X-ray

Your patient, Mr. Keller, is scheduled for posterior-anterior (PA) and lateral chest X-rays. Since he's ambulatory, he'll go to the X-ray department for the procedure. Although you won't be there to help him, you can prepare him for the procedure before he goes.

Don't neglect this preparation, even if he's had routine chest X-rays before. He may not have understood why. To teach him about X-rays, follow these guidelines:
• Tell him why the doctor's ordered X-rays, if possible.
• Explain the procedure. Tell him that the X-ray technician will take X-rays from the back and the side of his chest. For best results, the technician will ask the patient to stand with his hands on his hips for PA X-rays, and with his hands above his head for lateral X-rays.
• Describe the equipment he'll see. Remember, he may become apprehensive when he sees the large, unfamiliar machinery.
• Assure him that he'll receive only a small amount of radiation, and that the procedure's entirely safe. Explain that others in the room will shield themselves from the radiation because they're exposed to many X-rays each day.
• Is your patient a woman? Ask her when she had her last menstrual period. If there's any chance she's pregnant, ask the X-ray technician to shield the patient's uterus. Then, advise the patient of this special precaution.
• Warn the patient that the X-ray plate will feel cold.
• Warn him that he'll hear thudding sounds as the X-ray plates are changed.
• Encourage questions, and answer them completely and frankly.
• Ask him to remove jewelry and any other metal objects he's wearing above his waist. Explain that the metal will block the X-rays.
• Then, remove his clothing from the waist up and dress him in a hospital gown (or an X-ray gown, according to hospital policy). Tie the gown in the back, not the front. *Note:* Don't use a gown with metal snaps, because the snaps may show up on the X-rays and look like abnormalities.
• Tell your patient to stand erect during the procedure and to inhale deeply and hold his breath at the technician's request.

Helping with a portable X-ray machine

1 *What if your patient's too weak for a trip to the X-ray department? The doctor may order a chest X-ray taken with a portable machine, even though it can X-ray only the anterior-posterior view. Here's what you should do to help:*

Prepare the patient as you would for a standard X-ray in the X-ray department (see above).

Then, raise the head of the bed as high as possible, or as high as the patient can tolerate comfortably. By sitting the patient upright, you'll assure a clearer X-ray by reducing the pressure of her abdominal contents on her diaphragm and other thoracic structures.

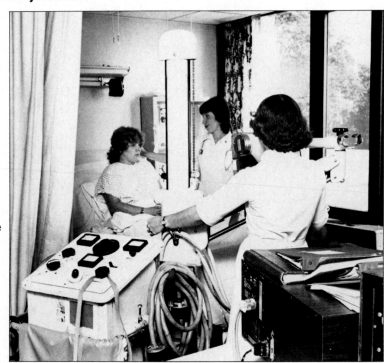

2 Remind the patient that the X-ray plate will feel cold on her back. Then, help the X-ray technician center it under the patient's back, as shown here.

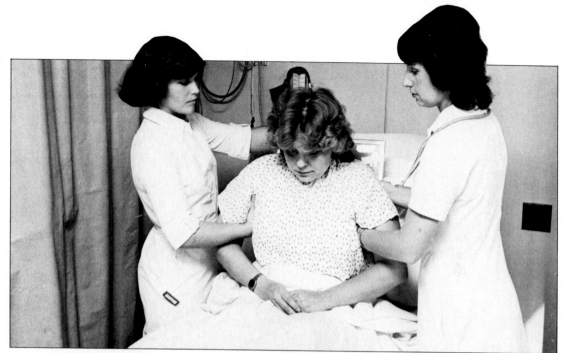

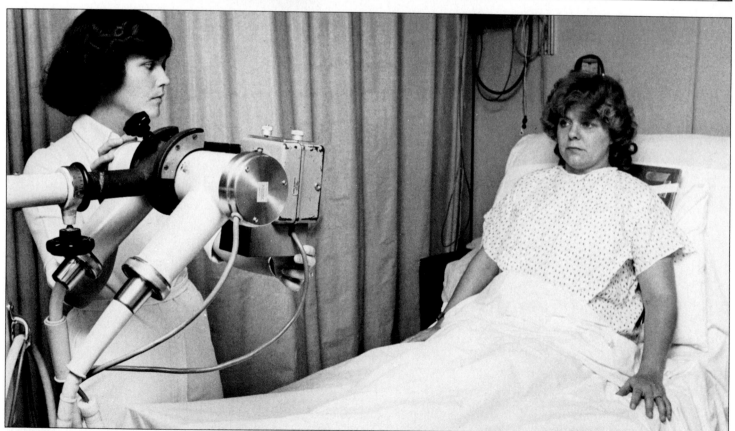

3 Urge the patient to inhale deeply and hold her breath when the technician tells her to. If necessary, repeat the technician's instructions for her. Your patient may respond better to the encouragement of a familiar person, like you.

Important: For safety, stand clear of the X-ray machine when X-rays are being taken—preferably behind a lead apron or out of the room. Make sure others do, too. This precaution's especially important for girls, and women of childbearing age.

Document the procedure on the patient's chart and in your nurses' notes. Be sure to note that the X-ray was taken with a portable X-ray machine, because the anterior-posterior view may distort the heart's size. Clearly document the patient's position, too. A recumbent position changes the heart's position in the thorax.

Radiography

Reading a normal X-ray

You can't learn to accurately read chest X-rays overnight. Skillful interpretation takes lots of experience. But with a little practice, you can learn to recognize some common signs of cardiopulmonary disease.

First, however, learn what a healthy heart and lung look like. To do this, study this X-ray. Notice the size, shape, and position of the heart and lungs, and their relationship to each other. Then, read the charts on page 55. They'll tell you how the radiologist identifies cardiac enlargement and pulmonary congestion.

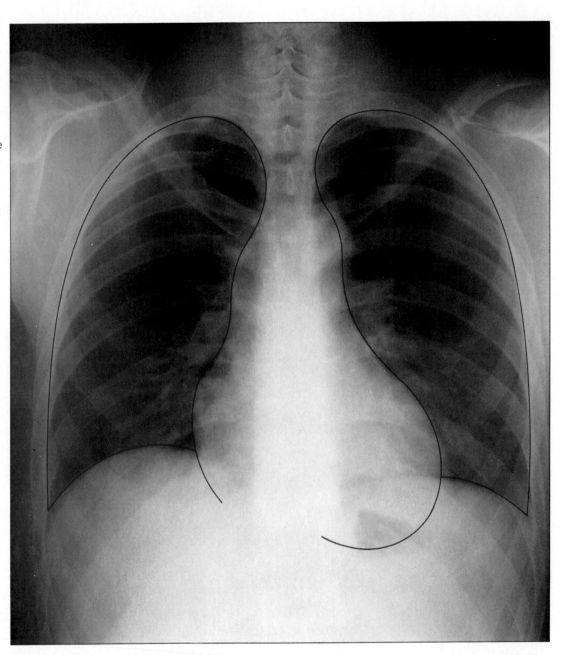

Estimating the cardiothoracic ratio

Since normal heart size varies among people, you may have a hard time deciding whether your patient suffers from cardiac enlargement just by looking at his X-rays. If you're lucky, you'll have an older chest X-ray to compare with a more recent one. This allows you to observe any changes. But if a recent X-ray is all that's available, you can judge the extent of cardiac enlargement by estimating the cardiothoracic ratio (size of patient's heart in comparison to his thoracic cage).

Normally, the thoracic cage is at least twice as wide as the heart when seen from the posterior-anterior (PA) view. To estimate the cardiothoracic ratio, use an X-ray taken from the PA view, like the one above. Measure the diameter of the cardiac silhouette at its widest point; then, compare it to the diameter of the thoracic cage at *its* widest point. If the heart fills more than half of the thoracic cage, suspect cardiac enlargement.

Keep in mind that the cardiothoracic ratio's only an estimate. With some patients, it can be misleading. A patient with chronic lung disease, for instance, may have an unusually large thorax, making his heart seem small by comparison. And a patient who failed to take a deep breath while the X-ray was taken may seem to have an enlarged heart.

Document your findings.

Recognizing cardiac enlargement

How can the radiologist tell if your patient's heart chambers are enlarged? In this chart, you'll learn about some of the clues he'll look for in the ventricles and left atrium. (Right atrial en-largement is rare, and usually doesn't show up on an X-ray.) *Note:* Although PA and lateral views are standard, the radiologist may study X-rays taken from other views, too.

Enlarged chamber	Posterior-anterior (PA) view	Lateral view
Left ventricle	Convex rounding of left cardiac border, with lateral, boot-shaped extension of lower left border	Posterior bulge of left ventricle
Right ventricle	Displacement of pulmonary artery toward left cardiac border	Anterior bulge near pulmonary artery
Left atrium	Lateral extension of right cardiac border	Posterior bulge at level of left atrium

Recognizing pulmonary congestion

When the heart malfunctions, the lungs may suffer, too. If the heart can't maintain adequate cardiac output, fluid backs up in the lungs, causing congestion. X-rays taken from the posterior-anterior (PA) view can help the radiologist evaluate respiratory conditions causing lung congestion. He'll also consult the patient's history before making a diagnosis.

Keep in mind that an X-ray may show evidence of all these conditions. That's one reason why correctly interpreting X-rays is so difficult.

Respiratory condition	X-ray findings (PA view)
Chronic pulmonary hypertension	• Antler-shaped cloudiness above base of heart caused by dilated pulmonary arteries
Alveolar edema	• Diffuse butterfly-shaped or puffy cloudiness in central lung field
Interstitial edema	• Linear, lacy, or honeycomb-shaped cloudiness that spreads peripherally and superiorly in lung field • Opaque, random lines in central areas, or opaque lines perpendicular to pleura in peripheral areas; indicating collection of fluid in lungs' interlobular septa

What's fluoroscopy?

As useful as they are, chest X-rays don't always present conclusive evidence that a patient has heart disease. To take a closer look at the patient's heart, the doctor may order a similar, but more comprehensive, procedure: cardiac fluoroscopy.

Using X-rays, cardiac fluoroscopy provides a constant image of the heart on a monitor screen. By examining the beating heart from many directions, the doctor can identify structural damage, examine heart wall movement, and assess prosthetic valve function. Fluoroscopy may also help him evaluate these conditions:
• aortic stenosis and insufficiency
• pericardial effusion
• cardiac calcifications
• heart chamber enlargement
• ventricular aneurysm.

Fluoroscopy's usually accompanied by a cardiac series, or barium swallow. While he's being X-rayed, the patient swallows a barium solution, which coats his esophagus. The coating highlights any deviations in the contour of the esophagus, which may be caused by left atrial enlargement. The barium coating may also make abnormalities of the aortic arch more easily visible.

At some hospitals, fluoroscopic findings are preserved on film, so the doctor can review them later. This process is called cinefluoroscopy. But if cinefluoroscopy isn't available in your hospital, individual fluoroscopic views may be recorded on spot films.

Fluoroscopy has one major disadvantage: it exposes the patient to 15 to 20 times more radiation than a chest X-ray. As a result, fluoroscopy may be contraindicated for some patients: pregnant women, for example. An alternative diagnostic procedure, such as echocardiography, may provide the doctor with enough information about your patient's heart without radiation risks.

Radiography

When your patient undergoes fluoroscopy

Let's say your patient's scheduled for fluoroscopy. A technician will probably perform the procedure in the X-ray department, although he may perform it in the ICU instead, if your hospital has a portable fluoroscopy unit. You're responsible for preparing the patient before the procedure and caring for him after it. Do you know what to do?

First, discuss fluoroscopy with him and answer his questions. Explain that the procedure's much like an X-ray, except that it produces a moving picture of the heart instead of a still picture. Also, inform your patient that this procedure exposes him to more radiation than an ordinary chest X-ray does, but that the additional amount isn't considered harmful.

In addition, tell him:
• why the doctor's ordered the test.
• what the equipment looks like. (Use the photo on this page as a guide.)
• what to expect during the test. For example, tell him that the room will be darkened during the procedure. To X-ray the heart from several angles, the technician will ask him to lie on his back and turn occasionally. Warn him that he may hear thudding noises when X-ray plates are changed.
• why he may be asked to swallow barium at the end of the procedure.
• what barium tastes like. Most likely, he won't find it unpalatable—in fact, it may be pleasantly flavored. But tell him to expect a chalky consistency, like milk of magnesia.

Before the patient leaves his room, remove his clothing from the waist up and help him into a hospital or X-ray gown. Remove any metal objects he's wearing on his upper body; for example, jewelry. Make sure his gown fastens with ties, not metal snaps.

After the procedure, the patient may resume his normal activities. However, if he was given a barium swallow, he'll need a cathartic to help pass the barium. Check your hospital's policy for guidelines.

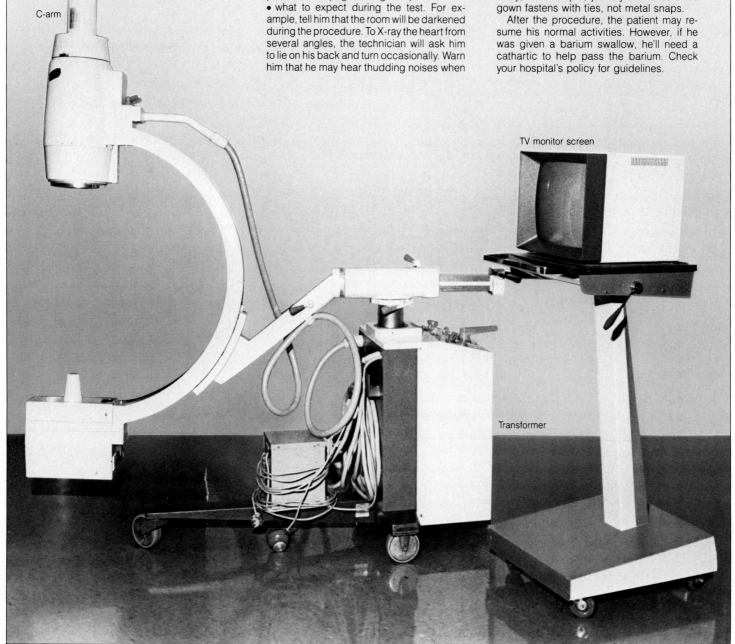

C-arm

TV monitor screen

Transformer

Learning about myocardial hot-spot imaging

You remember Lola Burton, a 59-year-old housewife. You cared for her about a year ago, after she had an acute myocardial infarction (MI). Now she's back in the ICU again. The diagnosis: a suspected myocardial infarction.

You see that Mrs. Burton's scheduled for myocardial hot-spot imaging. Do you know enough about the procedure to tell her why the doctor's ordered it? Can you tell her what the test will be like, and answer her questions about it? If not, read on.

Finding the hot spot

Myocardial hot-spot imaging requires intravenous injection of technetium pyrophosphate, a chemical compound that's tagged with a small amount of radioactive material. This compound circulates in your patient's bloodstream without hurting her.

Newly damaged heart tissue collects large amounts of the radioactive compound, causing a so-called *hot spot,* which can be detected by a special gamma scanner machine. Detection of a hot spot not only confirms a recent myocardial infarction, it distinguishes recent myocardial damage from old damage (which doesn't produce a hot spot). What's more, it pinpoints the damaged area.

Just how reliable is the procedure? In most cases, it's highly reliable when performed within three days of the infarction. However, some conditions may produce false positives; for example:
• ventricular aneurysm
• lung neoplasm
• recent electrical shock (for example, from a defibrillator) that may have damaged heart muscle.

Confirming the diagnosis

Why not use conventional tests, such as a 12-lead EKG, to confirm the diagnosis? Because for some patients, these tests aren't conclusive.

Mrs. Burton is an example.

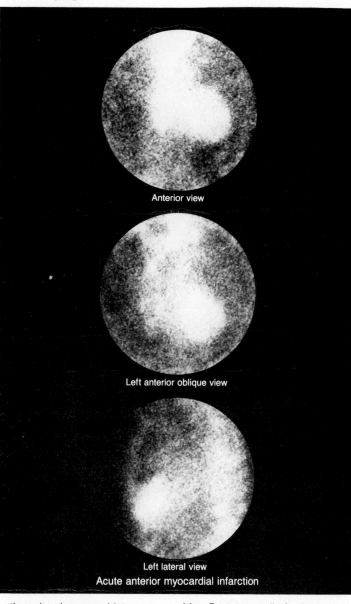

Anterior view

Left anterior oblique view

Left lateral view

Acute anterior myocardial infarction

Let's review her case history. While standing on a stepladder changing a light bulb, she lost consciousness and fell. Discovered by a neighbor, Mrs. Burton's now being treated for a broken arm, multiple contusions, and, possibly, myocardial infarction.

Myocardial infarction's certainly a reasonable diagnosis. After all, Mrs. Burton's had an MI before. What's more, her EKG shows an arrhythmia, and her cardiac enzyme level is high. And even though she can't remember the fall itself, Mrs. Burton recalls feeling chest discomfort that day. (She hoped it was just indigestion.)

Today, Mrs. Burton still has chest pain. Is the pain caused by a new myocardial infarction, as her cardiac enzyme level suggests? Or, is it caused by musculoskeletal bruising suffered during the fall?

The doctor can't be sure. Although Mrs. Burton's EKG *is* irregular, it may reflect past, not recent, heart damage. Pinpointing the problem's essential. Myocardial hot-spot imaging may provide the answer.

Preparing the patient

You won't do any of this procedure yourself, but you can make sure Mrs. Burton knows just what to expect. Tell her that a doctor or specially trained technician will inject a radioactive substance into a vein, in front of her elbow (antecubital fossa). Explain that the amount of radioactivity is very small—less than what she'd receive from a chest X-ray. Assure her that, except for brief discomfort from the needle, the entire procedure will be painless.

After the injection, she'll wait approximately 90 minutes before the scanning begins. This allows her kidneys to clear the radioactive substance from her bloodstream, which is necessary before the scanner can detect the tracer in her heart muscle.

Then, she'll be taken to the X-ray unit, where the doctor will position her flat on her back under the scanner. Describe the scanning machinery for her, so it won't frighten her when she sees it for the first time.

With the scanner, the doctor will take pictures of her heart from three different views. He'll take two views while she's on her back, and the third while she's on her left side. (For examples of these views, see the photos on the left.) Each scanning will take about 10 minutes. Tell her to remain still and breathe normally while each view's being taken. However, she may talk and move between views.

After the procedure, Mrs. Burton may resume whatever activities her condition permits. Later, after the doctor's discussed the test results with her, answer any questions she has.

Note: Another type of myocardial imaging, perfusion (or cold spot) imaging, uses thallium to identify areas of poor blood perfusion within the heart muscle. Because this test is, in many cases, performed along with an exercise EKG (stress test), we'll discuss it in the cardiac rehabilitation section.

Sonic tests

You may not realize it, but you're already familiar with sonic tests. Every time you listen to your patient's heart sounds with a stethoscope, you're performing one. In the following pages, you'll learn about two other sonic tests: phonocardiography and echocardiography.

Both of these tests use sound waves, but in very different ways. Phonocardiography records heart sounds, which are sound waves generated by the heart itself. Echocardiography, on the other hand, records the inaudible echos of ultrasonic waves as they bounce off the patient's heart. These ultrasonic waves are both generated and received by a special transducer placed on the patient's chest. When they're interpreted, the echos provide detailed and accurate information about the heart's size, position, density, and elasticity.

Want to learn more? Read the next few pages.

Learning about phonocardiography

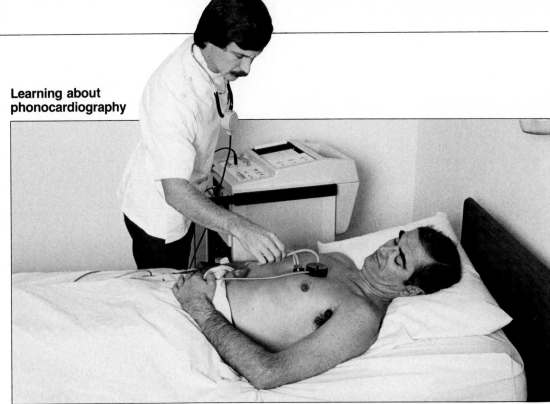

Have you ever auscultated a patient's heart and been confused by abnormal or unusual heart sounds? If so, you're not alone. Heart sounds can be very difficult to interpret, even for cardiac specialists. That's why phonocardiography's so valuable. By graphically reproducing those same heart sounds, it allows the doctor to examine them visually and interpret them more accurately.

To run a phonocardiograph, a skilled technician places microphones at the standard heart-auscultation locations on the patient's chest. A transducer in each microphone picks up heart sounds, amplifies them, converts them to electrical impulses, and transmits them to a recorder. The recorder then produces a graph (see the illustrations shown below). Such a graph helps the doctor:
• time events in your patient's cardiac cycle, including systolic time intervals.
• distinguish murmurs, gallop rhythms, and other abnormal heart sounds.

Note: A phonocardiograph can't tell the doctor much about the *cause* of abnormal heart sounds. As a result, phonocardiograms are nearly always accompanied by another diagnostic procedure; for example, an EKG or apexcardiogram (ACG).

Reading a phonocardiogram

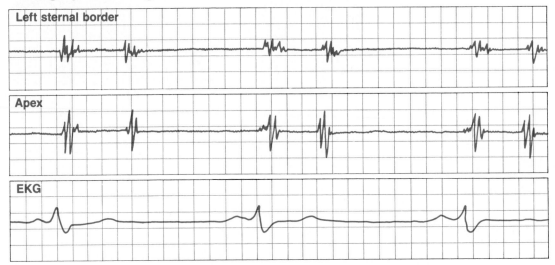

The waveforms you see on a phonocardiogram vary, depending on exactly where the microphone's placed. In this illustration, the first phonocardiograph waveform was recorded at the heart's left sternal border; the second at its apex. The EKG waveform shows how the phonocardiogram's waveforms relate to the cardiac cycle.

**Preparing your patient
for a phonocardiogram**

Mr. White's scheduled for a phonocardio-gram. *You* know it's a simple procedure, but does *he*? You can prepare him by telling him about the proce-dure. Here are some questions he's apt to ask, as well as an-swers you can give.

Patient's question	Your answer
What's a phonocardiogram? Sounds scary! I can hardly pronounce it!	A phonocardiogram's a simple, completely painless procedure with a long name. *Phono* simply means sound; *cardiogram* means a recording of your heart's activity that's drawn on graph paper. A phonocardiogram, then, is just a recording of your heart sounds.
How's this recording made?	A skilled technician will place one or more small microphones on your chest and secure them with chest straps. These microphones will pick up the sounds your heart makes as it beats. Then, a recording machine will draw a series of waves representing your heart sounds. These waves help the doctor learn how well your heart's functioning. At the same time, the technician will run an EKG. Do you under-stand how EKGs work? (If Mr. White's not sure, teach him about EKGs, using the guidelines on page 39.)
Can the technician perform this test in my room?	No, because your room's too noisy. Any background noise can distort the recording. You'll go to a special room that's quiet and comfortable for this procedure.
What do *I* do?	During the procedure, the technician may ask you to change posi-tion, perform isometric (muscle-clenching) exercises, or do certain breathing maneuvers. Your doctor can tell a lot about your heart by studying how your heart sounds change when you move as instructed. To study other heart sounds, your doctor may also want you to inhale a gas called amyl nitrite. This gas, which has a slightly sweet odor, may affect the way your heart sounds, too. Don't be alarmed if you feel dizzy or flushed, or if you experience a rapid heartbeat for a short time after inhaling the gas. But report any unusual sensations to the doctor or technician.
Do I need any special prepara-tion or care for this procedure?	Not really. You can eat normally and continue your usual activities, both before and after the procedure. But if your chest is hairy, the technician may shave it before applying the microphones. To assure a clear phonocardiogram, the microphones must stick closely to the skin.
When will I find out my test results?	The doctor will discuss them with you as soon as he's finished examining the phonocardiogram. Most of the time, this takes a day or two. Then, if you have any questions, I'll try to answer them for you.

Sonic tests

Echocardiography: Why it's used

The doctor may order echocardiography for your patient because it's:
• noninvasive.
• painless.
• without contraindications.
• highly reliable for evaluating certain cardiac structure abnormalities.
• convenient. May be performed at bedside, if necessary.

Echocardiography can help the doctor assess:
• heart chamber size.
• heart valve motion.
• septal wall motion.
• left ventricular wall thickness and motion.
• left ventricular volume.

Echocardiography can help the doctor diagnose:
• valvular disorders, for example, mitral valve prolapse; and mitral, tricuspid, or pulmonic valve insufficiency.
• congenital disorders, such as atrioseptal defect.
• pericardial effusion or cardiac tamponade.
• subvalvular stenosis.
• cardiac tumors.
• prosthetic valve malfunctions.

Understanding echocardiography

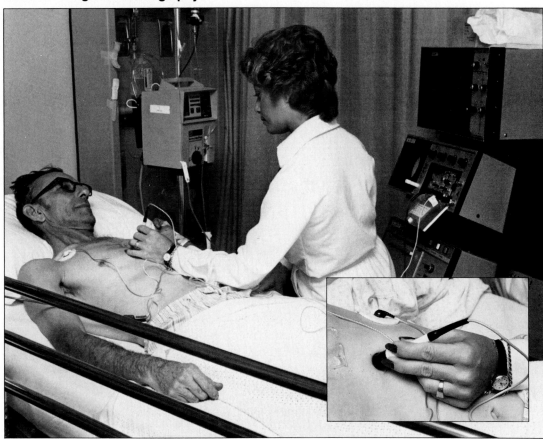

Do you understand echocardiography well enough to explain it to your patient? If not, this background information will help.

To perform echocardiography, a technician places the patient on his back. Then, she applies conductive jelly to the third or fourth intercostal space to the left of the sternum, and places a dime-sized transducer on it. This transducer acts as both a transmitter of ultrasonic waves, and a receiver of the returning echos.

Why is the transducer placed at the third or fourth intercostal space? Because either of these locations provides an *acoustical window* that avoids lung and bone tissue. (As you know, ultrasound travels poorly through bone and lung tissue.)

When the transducer's in place, the technician systematically angles it to direct ultrasonic waves at different parts of the patient's heart (see inset). The returning echos are displayed on the oscilloscope and recorded on a readout strip.

Depending on its depth and thickness, each part of the patient's heart returns a specific echo pattern. And because the transducer emits 1,000 ultrasonic waves per second, the echo pattern reflects continuous cardiac motion.

For another perspective on the heart, the technician may position the transducer differently; for example, beneath the xiphoid process or directly above the sternum. Or, she may reposition the patient on his left side for a left lateral view.

With this background, you can teach the patient all he needs to know about echocardiography. Remember to explain it to him in words he can understand. Assure him that the procedure's painless and risk-free. As you talk with him, don't forget these additional points:
• In most cases, the procedure will take only 15 minutes, unless it's accompanied by other diagnostic tests: for example, an apexcardiogram (ACG), pulse wave tracings, or an EKG.
• The technician may darken the room, so she can see the oscilloscope screen better.
• The technician may ask the patient to perform breathing exercises, so she can record heart function under different conditions.
• The technician may ask the patient to inhale amyl nitrate, a gas with a slightly sweet odor. Then, she'll record the resulting changes in heart sounds. Warn the patient about possible side effects, such as dizziness, tachycardia, or flushing. Tell him that these feelings will pass quickly, but urge him to report them anyway.
• Movement may distort the test results. Instruct the patient to lie still throughout the procedure.

After the procedure, the patient may resume normal activity. Remember to follow up on test results and answer any questions the patient has about them.

Reading an echocardiogram

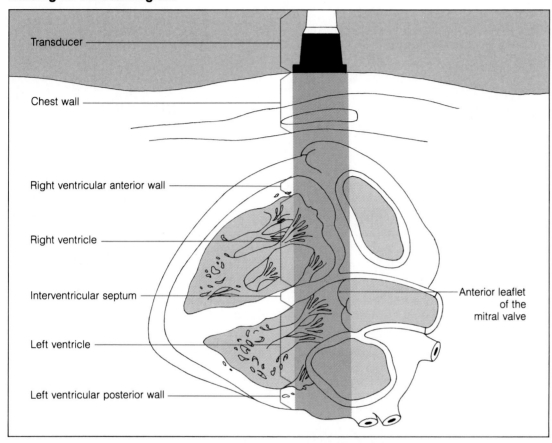

Transducer

Chest wall

Right ventricular anterior wall

Right ventricle

Interventricular septum

Left ventricle

Left ventricular posterior wall

Anterior leaflet
of the
mitral valve

The illustrations on this page
show how an echocardiogram
represents the heart's structure.
First, look at the illustration to
the left. It shows the ultrasonic
transducer placed in a standard
aiming direction. The shaded
area beneath the transducer
identifies the cardiac structures
that intercept and reflect the
transducer's ultrasonic waves.

Note: Because they're continuous membrane layers, the
endocardium, epicardium, and
pericardium aren't shown in
this illustration.

Now, look at the tracing and
the simplified illustration at
the bottom of the page. Together, they show you how the
echocardiogram depicts these
cardiac structures.

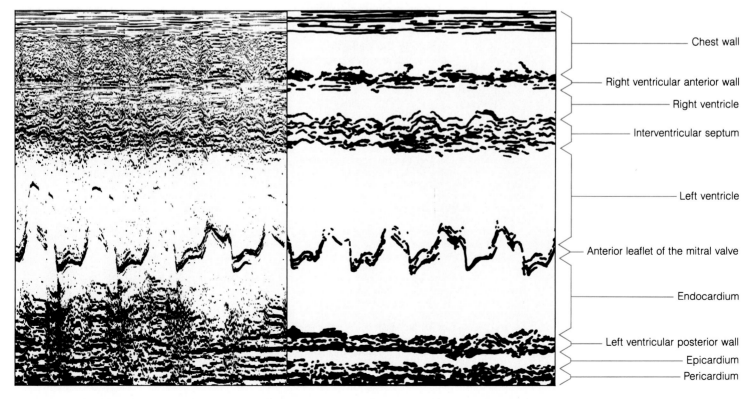

Chest wall

Right ventricular anterior wall

Right ventricle

Interventricular septum

Left ventricle

Anterior leaflet of the mitral valve

Endocardium

Left ventricular posterior wall

Epicardium

Pericardium

Pulse wave tracings

Let's say the doctor wants to assess the timing of mechanical events in the cardiac cycle. To do this, he may order pulse wave tracings, a painless, risk-free diagnostic procedure.

Pulse wave tracings record low-frequency, soundless vibrations from the jugular vein, the carotid artery, or the heart's apex. These vibrations reflect the heart's pulsations during diastole and systole.

What do pulse wave tracings tell the doctor about your patient's condition? How's the procedure performed? What does your patient need to know about it? For answers, read these pages.

What pulse wave tracings show

By themselves, pulse wave tracings usually don't provide enough information to make an accurate diagnosis. But when compared with other diagnostic tests, they often supply valuable supplementary information, as indicated here.

Carotid artery tracings may help identify:
● aortic valve disease.
● idiopathic hypertrophic sub-aortic stenosis.
● left ventricular failure.
● hypertension.

Jugular vein tracings may help identify:
● right-sided heart failure, causing increased right atrial pressure.
● tricuspid valve disorders.

Precordial pulsation tracings (apexcardiography) may help identify:
● heart sounds.
● ventricular enlargement, infarction, and/or ischemia.
● ventricular aneurysm.
● pericarditis.

Taking jugular and carotid pulse wave tracings

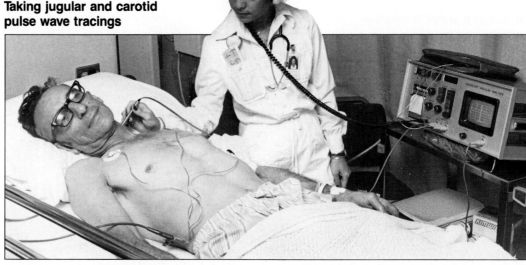

In most hospitals, a skilled technician records jugular and carotid pulse wave tracings. Here's how:

First, she'll place the patient on his back, with his head turned to one side and his neck slightly hyperextended. To make the jugular vein or carotid artery more accessible, she'll elevate his head slightly.

Next, she'll place a sensor over either the jugular vein or carotid artery, 1 to 2 inches below the jaw. If the sensor's attached to a suction cup, she'll simply apply it to the patient's neck. If it's not attached to a suction cup, she'll hold it gently against the patient's neck with her fingers, as shown above. But for prolonged recordings, she may secure the sensor against the patient's neck with a pediatric blood-pressure cuff inflated to less than 20 mm Hg. *Note:* She may record additional jugular tracings from the supraclavicular area.

Pulse wave tracings look like the examples on the opposite page. A carotid tracing's more distinct (and easier to interpret) than a jugular tracing, because the carotid artery has such a strong pulse. The carotid artery's pulse is so strong, in fact, that it may interfere with a jugular pulse wave tracing.

The technician nearly always runs a simultaneous phonocardiogram or lead II EKG. These simultaneous recordings help clarify the timing of events in the cardiac cycle.

PATIENT TEACHING

Teaching the patient about pulse wave tracings

Is your patient scheduled for either a carotid or a jugular pulse wave test? If so, you needn't give him any special care beforehand. He may continue to eat and receive medication as usual. But, do take time to explain the procedure to him and answer his questions. As you talk, be sure to cover these points:
● *Why the doctor's ordered the test,* if that information's available.
● *How the test will feel.* Assure him that it's entirely painless. But warn him that he may hear a harsh sound when the sensor's placed over his carotid artery.
● *How long the test will last.* In most cases, it takes about a half hour, unless other tests are performed at the same time or the tracing is continuous.
● *How the patient will be positioned.* Explain that he'll lie on his back with his neck slightly hyper-extended. For an arterial pulse wave tracing, the technician will want him to turn his head away

from the carotid artery that's being tested.
● *How the transducer will be held in place.* If the technician plans to secure it with a pediatric pressure cuff, assure the patient that the cuff won't be uncomfortable, or restrict his breathing or blood flow.
● *What he'll do during the procedure.* Tell him to lie quietly, without talking. The technician may ask him to hold his breath occasionally, so breathing sounds don't interfere with recording.
● *What other tests will be performed at the same time.* Most likely, the technician will also run a phonocardiogram. Make sure the patient understands this procedure as well. (For tips on preparing him for a phonocardiogram, see page 58.)
● *How the test will affect the patient's activity.* Tell him that he won't need any special care after the test, and that he may resume his usual activities immediately.

Reading a carotid pulse wave tracing

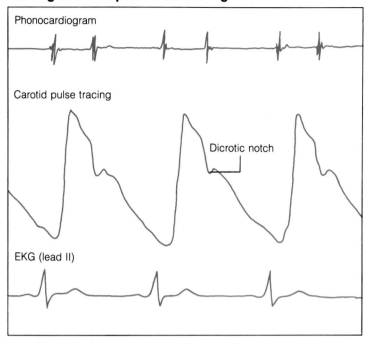

Phonocardiogram

Carotid pulse tracing

Dicrotic notch

EKG (lead II)

This illustration shows a normal carotid pulse wave tracing, accompanied by a simultaneous phonocardiogram and a simultaneous lead II EKG. Note the prominent dicrotic notch on the carotid pulse tracing. This tells you when the aortic valve closes in relation to other mechanical events.

Reading a jugular pulse wave tracing

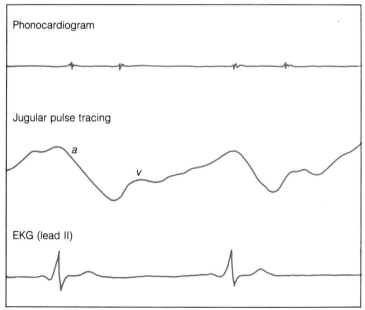

Phonocardiogram

Jugular pulse tracing

a

v

EKG (lead II)

This illustration shows a normal jugular pulse wave tracing, accompanied by a simultaneous phonocardiogram and a simultaneous lead II EKG. The most important segments of the jugular tracing are the *a* wave and the *v* wave. The *a* wave indicates active atrial contraction; the *v* wave indicates atrial filling, and bulging of the tricuspid valve into the atrium during ventricular systole.

Preparing the patient for apexcardiography

As you know, an apexcardiogram (ACG) is a pulse wave tracing of low-frequency precordial pulsations. The doctor may order it to evaluate left ventricular heart function, or to help him identify heart sounds.

Like other pulse wave tracings, the ACG is simple and painless. Your patient needs no special care, either before or after the procedure. But, you should prepare him for the procedure, using these guidelines:

• Explain the procedure, including why the doctor's ordered it for him.
• Assure him that the procedure's risk-free and painless.
• Prepare the patient for a simultaneous EKG. Make sure he understands EKGs by reviewing with him the information on page 39.
• Explain that the technician will record his heartbeat by strapping a sensor to his chest. She'll probably take recordings while he's lying on his left side and when he's lying flat on his back.
• Advise him that the technician may ask him to do special exercises or breathing maneuvers during the procedure. This lets her record his heartbeat under different conditions. *Note:* The doctor may order a stress test between ACG recordings. If so, be sure to explain this to the patient. (For details on stress testing, see the section on cardiac rehabilitation.)
• Remind the patient not to talk or move during the test, unless the technician asks him to do so. This helps assure a clear recording.

Reading an ACG

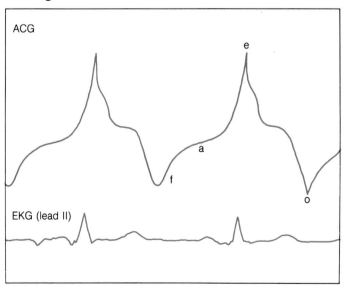

ACG

e

a

f

o

EKG (lead II)

This illustration shows a normal apexcardiogram (ACG), accompanied by a simultaneous lead II EKG. Here's what the ACG waveform tells you about the cardiac cycle:
a point: Atrial systole; ventricular filling
e point: Ventricular systole; aortic valve opens
o point: Mitral valve opens (approximate time)
o to f: Rapid ventricular filling
f to e: Slow ventricular filling

Invasive tests

So far, all the tests we've discussed in this book are noninvasive. In the following pages, we'll take a look at some tests that require catheter insertion directly into the heart's chambers.

To begin, let's define the term *cardiac catheterization*. We'll use this term in its broadest sense, to mean inserting a catheter directly into either the right or left side of the heart.

Either side of the heart may be catheterized to determine blood pressure and blood flow in the heart's chambers, to withdraw blood samples, or to record pictures of the heart (angiography). In addition, the right side of the heart may be catheterized to obtain an EKG directly from the right atrium. One of these tests is called the His bundle EKG (HBE).

Invasive tests differ in purpose, as well as in the ways they represent the heart and its activity. Angiography, for example, produces the heart's image on X-ray film. The HBE, on the other hand, represents the heart's electrical activity on an electrocardiogram. But despite their differences, these invasive tests share similar techniques for patient preparation and care.

What do you need to know about cardiac catheterization to give your patient complete care, both before and after the procedure? To find out, read the following pages.

Learning about cardiac catheterization basics

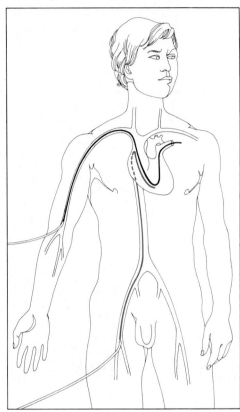

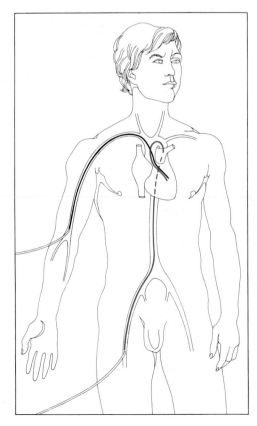

As you know, a doctor can catheterize either the left or right side of the heart. In some cases, he may catheterize more than one chamber at a time. He'll do the procedure in the catheterization (cath) lab.

How does he insert the catheter? Let's consider right-sided catheterization first. Look at the first illustration on the left. Most likely, the doctor will insert the catheter into a median cubital or basilic vein, using a cutdown procedure. However, he may choose a femoral vein instead, depending on his preference and the patient's condition. Then, guided by fluoroscopy, he'll pass the catheter through the vein into the right atrium. (If he's using the femoral vein, he'll pass the catheter through the inferior vena cava instead, as the illustration shows.)

If the doctor's assessing cardiac conduction, with a His bundle EKG (HBE) for example, he'll pass the catheter tip across the tricuspid valve into the right ventricle. But, for most other diagnostic tests, he'll continue to pass the catheter through the right ventricle, across the pulmonary valve, and into the pulmonary artery. From there, he can collect blood samples, measure pulmonary artery wedge pressure, and assess cardiac output.

Note: The doctor may perform left heart studies from the right side by puncturing the atrial septum. This procedure's called transseptal catheterization.

Now, suppose the doctor's catheterizing the *left* side of the patient's heart. Look at the second illustration. As you see, the procedure's much the same as it is for right-sided catheterization, except that the doctor uses an artery instead of a vein. To do this, he may perform an arteriotomy in the antecubital fossa, or percutaneously puncture a femoral artery. Then, he'll advance the catheter through the aorta and into the left ventricle, while monitoring the catheter's progress on the fluoroscope.

While the catheter's in the left ventricle, the doctor may perform angiography by injecting a contrast medium (indocyanine green dye) into the ventricle. This dye permits him to see the ventricle and the aorta clearly on the fluoroscope and on X-rays.

Note: If the doctor takes a motion picture of the heart, the procedure's called *cineangiography*.

Angiography of the left ventricle helps the doctor diagnose:
- left ventricular enlargement.
- aortic stenosis and regurgitation.
- aortic root enlargement.
- mitral regurgitation.
- intracardiac shunt.
- aneurysm.

The doctor may use a similar procedure to perform coronary arteriography (also called coronary angiography, or coronary cineangiography). To do this, he injects dye directly into one or more of the patient's coronary arteries. This procedure helps him locate coronary artery obstructions.

After performing diagnostic tests on either side of the heart, the doctor will remove the catheter, apply a dressing to the insertion site, and return the patient to your care.

Acquainting your patient with the catheterization lab

Imagine this: you're lying flat on your back on a rock-hard surface. Someone's glued wires all over your body. Heavy machines dangle from the ceiling, making you worry that they'll fall at any minute and crush you. The room seems lit only by the glow from tv screens. You hear mysterious thudding sounds, but you can't tell where they're coming from. While you lie there helplessly, masked people bustle around you. You're trapped in a nightmare—or so it seems.

Sound horrendous? Well, that's exactly how your patient may feel during cardiac catheterization, unless you prepare

him carefully. Remember, he'll be fully conscious. And, because the procedure may last for hours, he'll have plenty of time to fear the worst.

Don't keep your patient guessing. Sit down and describe the procedure to him ahead of time. (For guidelines, read the following page.) Then, using the photo on this page as a guide, describe all the strange equipment he'll see: monitors, cameras, fluoroscopes, electrocardiographs, and so on. By telling your patient what to expect, you spare him needless anxiety.

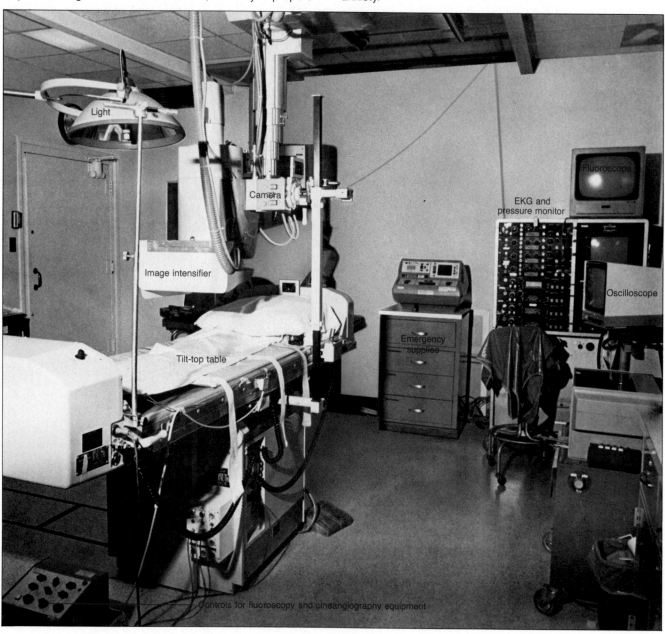

Invasive tests

Preparing your patient for cardiac catheterization

As you know, the doctor will do cardiac catheterization in a special lab, or in the ICU (if your hospital has a portable fluoroscopy unit). Your responsibility is to care for the patient before and after the procedure.

Begin preparing the patient as soon as he's scheduled for the procedure. To do so, follow these guidelines:

• Temporarily discontinue cardioactive medications, such as digoxin, if the doctor orders.

• If the patient's scheduled for *right-sided* heart catheterization, discontinue anticoagulant therapy, according to the doctor's orders. Doing so reduces the risk of complications from venous bleeding.

• But, if the patient's scheduled for *left-sided* heart catheterization, continue or begin anticoagulant therapy, according to the doctor's orders. By doing this, you reduce the risk of clotting at the catheter tip, a common problem with arterial catheters.

• Explain the procedure thoroughly to the patient and answer his questions. Tell him he may wear his glasses and dentures (if he has any) during the procedure. (For guidelines on teaching the patient about the procedure, read the information in the box below.)

• Make sure the patient's signed a consent form.

• If the procedure's scheduled for early morning, don't let your patient eat or drink anything for breakfast. But, if it's scheduled for late morning, the doctor may permit a clear liquid breakfast. These precautions reduce the risk of vomiting during the procedure, especially if the patient undergoes angiography.

• If your patient's scheduled for angiography, ask him if he has any allergies, especially an allergy to fish or iodine. If so, tell the doctor at once. Since the dye used for angiography has an iodine base, such a patient may suffer anaphylaxis when the dye's injected.

• If the insertion site's at the patient's groin or another hairy area, shave his skin. But first, ask the patient's permission and explain why shaving's necessary.

• If the doctor orders, establish an I.V. line of 5% dextrose in water or normal saline solution at keep-vein-open (KVO) rate. This will allow the doctor to give antiarrhythmic medication quickly, if necessary.

Teaching your patient about cardiac catheterization

Michael Addis, a 66-year-old accountant, is worried. His doctor's just scheduled him for cardiac angiography, and explained the risks to him. "I don't like the idea of having something stuck into my heart," he tells you. "My wife's sister had angiography, and said it was terrible. I'm not looking forward to this."

What can you tell Mr. Addis? You know that angiography involves some risks, like any procedure requiring cardiac catheterization. You also know that some patients find the procedure unpleasant. However, you can assure Mr. Addis that the doctor and the other health-care professionals in the cath lab perform cardiac catheterizations every day, and rarely encounter complications. In addition, you can tell him that most patients don't find angiography painful—in fact, some even doze off for short periods of time during the procedure. But do prepare him to feel occasional discomfort; for example, a hot flash when the dye's injected.

Try to see the procedure from Mr. Addis' viewpoint. What exactly will he experience? Then, take him step by step through the procedure. Doing so should quickly relieve most of his fears.

Now, let's imagine you're talking to your patient. Here's what to tell him:

• "The doctor doesn't want you to eat or drink anything for 6 to 12 hours before the procedure. This will help keep you from feeling nauseated, as some patients do when the dye's injected."

• "Expect to be fully conscious during the procedure, although the doctor may order a mild sedative for you. The procedure will last 2 to 3 hours."

• "Before you leave your room to go to the cath lab, I'll help you into a hospital gown and ask you to urinate."

• "When you get to the cath lab, you may be strapped to a padded table. This will keep you from falling off the table when the doctor tilts it to view your heart from different angles."

• "The doctors and nurses in the cath lab will wear gowns, gloves, and masks, to protect you from infection."

• "You'll have electrodes on your chest, arms, and legs, so the doctor can run an EKG during the procedure. Don't be surprised if the nurse slips the gown from your arms to give the doctor easier access to your chest."

• "You'll also have an I.V. needle inserted in your arm, so the doctor can give you medication through an I.V. line, if necessary."

• "The doctor will choose an artery or vein in your arm or leg for catheter insertion. If the skin above the blood vessel is hairy, the nurse will shave it. Next, she'll clean the skin with an antiseptic."

• "Then, the doctor will inject an anesthetic into the insertion site. You may feel some discomfort when he does this, but the entire area will soon become numb."

• "When the area's completely numb, he'll insert a needle into the artery or vein, and pass the catheter through the needle into the blood vessel. Then, he'll remove the needle and advance the catheter up the blood vessel into the heart. As a guide, he'll watch the catheter's progress on a special television screen that's known as a fluoroscope. If the screen is close enough, you may watch it too, if you wish."

• "As the doctor advances the catheter through the blood vessel, you may feel pressure, but it won't be painful."

• "Don't worry if the doctor withdraws the catheter and repeats the procedure with another blood vessel. He'll do this if a vessel obstruction prevents him from advancing the catheter to the heart."

• "As the catheter enters your heart, you may feel fluttering or flip-flop sensations. Report these feelings to the doctor, but try not to let them frighten you. They're normal reactions."

• "When the catheter's in place, the doctor will inject a dye through it. This makes the heart show up clearly on both the fluoroscope and X-rays. You may feel a hot flash, a burning sensation, or nausea when the dye's injected, but these sensations should disappear quickly."

• "The doctor may ask you to cough or pant occasionally. This helps propel the dye through the heart, and encourages the heart to maintain its steady rhythm."

• "The doctor also may ask you to take deep breaths. This depresses your diaphragm, and helps the doctor see your heart better."

• "During the procedure, the doctor may place a clip on your nose and ask you to breathe into a mouthpiece. This allows him to test your lung function."

• "Don't be startled if you hear loud thudding sounds. These sounds occur as pictures are taken, or as X-ray plates are changed."

• "Tell the doctor or nurse if you feel any unusual sensation at any time during the procedure; for example, chest pain, lightheadedness, a fluttering sensation in the chest, itching, flushing, or tightness in the throat."

Caring for the patient after the procedure

After your patient returns from the catheterization lab, make him comfortable and watch him closely for complications. (To learn how to recognize and deal with the complications of cardiac catheterization, study the chart on pages 68 and 69.) Make these postprocedure actions part of your routine:

• Monitor the rate and rhythm of your patient's heart immediately after he returns, if this is hospital policy. If he's not on a continuous cardiac monitor, run a 12-lead EKG.

• Take his vital signs every 15 minutes, for at least an hour, or until they're stable. Then, continue to take them frequently, to make sure they remain stable.

Important: Reassure your patient that this is a routine procedure, so he doesn't become frightened.

• Regularly check the pressure bandage over the insertion site. The bandage should be dry and secure, but not tight enough to restrict blood flow below the site.

• Keep the patient's limb straight and immobile to discourage bleeding. Use a splint or arm board, if necessary.

• At least once every half hour, check the limb below the insertion site for pulse, color, warmth, and sensation. At the same time, ask the patient to wiggle the fingers or toes of that limb.

• See that the patient gets 6 to 24 hours of bed rest after the procedure, depending on hospital policy.

• If your patient has had angiography, monitor his fluid output carefully. He runs the risk of becoming dehydrated, because the contrast dye acts as a powerful diuretic.

• If you discontinued cardioactive or anticoagulant medication before the procedure, find out if the doctor wants you to resume it.

• Document all observations on the patient's chart and in your nurses' notes. Notify the doctor of any complications.

• Follow up on test results. After the doctor's informed the patient of the results, discuss them with the patient and answer any questions he has.

The His bundle EKG: Assessing cardiac conduction

So far, we've discussed cardiac catheterization procedures that visualize the heart by X-ray. But the His bundle EKG (one type of intracardiac electrophysiologic test) is different, because it produces an electrocardiogram. Unlike a 12-lead EKG, which picks up the heart's electrical signals as they reach the patient's skin, a His bundle EKG (HBE) directly measures the heart's electrical activity from the right side of the patient's heart.

To insert the multipolar catheter necessary for an HBE, the doctor first performs a cutdown procedure on a vein, usually the right femoral vein. (He may choose a basilic or median cubital vein instead, depending on his preference or the patient's condition.) Then, guided by fluoroscopy, he advances the catheter up the vein, through the inferior vena cava, and into the right side of the heart. When the catheter's in place across the tricuspid valve, he records signals from each pole (either simultaneously or sequentially) on an electrocardiogram. The electrocardiogram reflects electrical potentials from the right atrium and the right ventricle, including the bundle of His.

The doctor may also insert another multipolar catheter into the left femoral vein, and advance it through the inferior vena cava to the right atrium. This way, he can record electrical potential from the upper right atrium at the same time.

As the doctor takes the HBE recordings, he will also monitor the patient with a 12-lead EKG. Later, he'll compare the HBE and EKG tracings. (For an example of HBE and 12-lead EKG tracings, see the illustration below.) This comparison helps the doctor assess:
• the location and extent of a conduction system block.
• the type of arrhythmia.
• the need for medication to treat a cardiac arrhythmia or other conduction disorder.
• the effectiveness of an artificial pacemaker.

Examining a His bundle EKG (HBE) waveform

The HBE's major waves are called A, H, and V. The A wave represents low right atrial activity; the H wave represents His bundle activity; and the V wave represents right ventricular activity. As you see, the HBE waveform reflects the EKG waveform.

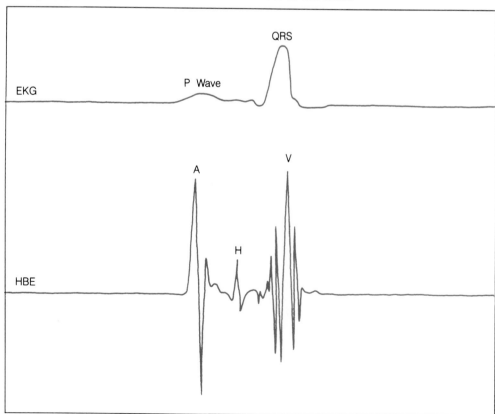

Invasive tests

Nurses' guide to cardiac catheterization complications

When your patient returns from the cath lab, do you know what complications to look for? Use this chart to review your skills.

As you know, cardiac catheterization imposes more risks than most other diagnostic tests. Although the possibility of complications is slight, some of the complications can be life-threatening. That's why you must watch your patient closely during the first 48 hours after the procedure.

Keep in mind that some complications are common to *both* left- and right-sided heart catheterization; others result only from catheterization of one side.

Note: An anaphylactic reaction to the contrast dye used for angiography may occur within 15 minutes of dye injection. Since this complication occurs in the cath lab, we haven't included it in this chart.

Possible complication of either left- or right-sided catheterization	Possible cause	Signs and symptoms	Nursing considerations
Myocardial infarction	• Emotional stress induced by procedure • Catheter tip dislodged blood clot, which traveled to a coronary artery (left-sided catheterization only)	• Chest pain, possibly radiating to left arm, back, and/or jaw • Cardiac arrhythmias • Diaphoresis, restlessness, and/or anxiety • Thready pulse • Temperature rise • Peripheral cyanosis, causing cool skin	• Call for a code team and begin CPR, if necessary. • Notify doctor. • Give oxygen and other drugs, as ordered. • Monitor patient's heart rate closely. • Document complication and treatment.
Arrhythmias	• Cardiac tissue irritated by catheter	• Irregular heartbeat • Irregular apical pulse • Palpitations	• Notify doctor. • Monitor patient continuously, as ordered. • Administer antiarrhythmic drugs, if ordered. • Document complication and treatment.
Cardiac tamponade	• Perforation of heart wall by catheter	• Arrhythmias • Increased heart rate • Decreased blood pressure • Chest pain • Diaphoresis • Cyanosis	• Notify doctor. • Give oxygen, if ordered. • Prepare patient for emergency surgery, if ordered. • Monitor patient continuously, as ordered. • Document complication and treatment.
Infection (systemic)	• Poor aseptic technique • Catheter contaminated during manufacturing process, storage, or use	• Fever • Increased pulse rate • Chills and tremors • Unstable blood pressure	• Notify doctor. • Collect samples of patient's urine, sputum, and blood for culture, as ordered. • Document complication and treatment.
Hypovolemia	• Diuresis from angiography dye	• Increased urine output • Hypotension	• Replace fluids by giving the patient one or two glasses of water every hour, or maintain I.V. at a rate of 150 to 200 ml/hour, as ordered. • Monitor fluid intake and output closely. • Document complication and treatment.
Hematoma, or blood loss at insertion site	• Bleeding at insertion site, from vein or artery damage	• Bloody dressing • Limb swelling • Decreased blood pressure • Increased heart rate	• Elevate limb and apply direct manual pressure. • When the bleeding's stopped, apply a pressure bandage. • If bleeding continues, or if vital signs are unstable, notify doctor. • Document complication and treatment.

Possible complication of either left- or right-sided catheterization	Possible cause	Signs and symptoms	Nursing considerations
Dye reaction	• Allergy to iodine base of angiography dye	• Fever • Agitation • Hives • Itching • Decreased urine output, indicating kidney failure	• Notify doctor. • Administer antihistamines to relieve itching, as ordered. • Adminiser diuretics to treat kidney failure, as ordered. • Monitor fluid intake and output closely. • Document complication and treatment.
Infection at insertion site	• Poor aseptic technique	• Swelling, warmth, redness, and soreness at site • Purulent discharge at site	• Obtain drainage sample for culture. • Clean site and apply antimicrobial ointment, if ordered. Cover site with sterile gauze pad. • Review and improve aseptic technique. • Document complication and treatment.

Possible complication of left-sided catheterization	Possible cause	Signs and symptoms	Nursing considerations
Arterial embolus or thrombus in limb	• Injury to artery during catheter insertion, causing blood clot • Catheter dislodged plaque from artery wall	• Slow or faint pulse distal to insertion site • Loss of warmth, sensation, and color in limb distal to insertion site	• Notify doctor. He may perform an arteriotomy and Fogarty catheterization to remove embolus or thrombus. • Protect affected limb from pressure. Keep it at room temperature and maintain in a level or slightly dependent position. • Administer vasodilators such as papaverine hydrochloride to relieve painful vasospasm, if ordered. • Document complication and treatment.
Cerebrovascular accident (CVA)	• Catheter tip dislodged blood clot or plaque, which traveled to brain	• Hemiplegia • Aphasia • Lethargy • Confusion, or decreased consciousness level	• Notify doctor. • Monitor vital signs closely. • Keep suctioning equipment nearby. • Give oxygen, as ordered. • Document complication and treatment.

Possible complication of right-sided catheterization	Possible cause	Signs and symptoms	Nursing considerations
Thrombophlebitis	• Vein damaged during catheter insertion	• Vein is hard, sore, cordlike, and warm to the touch. Vein may look like a red line above the catheter insertion site. • Swelling at site	• Elevate limb and apply warm, wet compresses. • Notify doctor. • Administer anticoagulant or fibrinolytic drugs, if ordered. • Document complication and treatment.
Pulmonary embolism	• Catheter tip dislodged blood clot or plaque, which traveled to lungs	• Shortness of breath • Hyperventilation • Increased heart rate • Chest pain	• Notify doctor. • Place patient in high Fowler's position. • Administer oxygen, if ordered. • Monitor vital signs. • Document complication and treatment.
Vagal response	• Vagus nerve endings irritated in sinoatrial (SA) node, atrial muscle tissue, or artrioventricular (AV) junction	• Hypotension • Decreased heart rate • Nausea	• Notify doctor. • Monitor heart rate closely. • Administer atropine, if ordered. • Keep patient supine and quiet. • Give liquids. • Document complication and treatment.

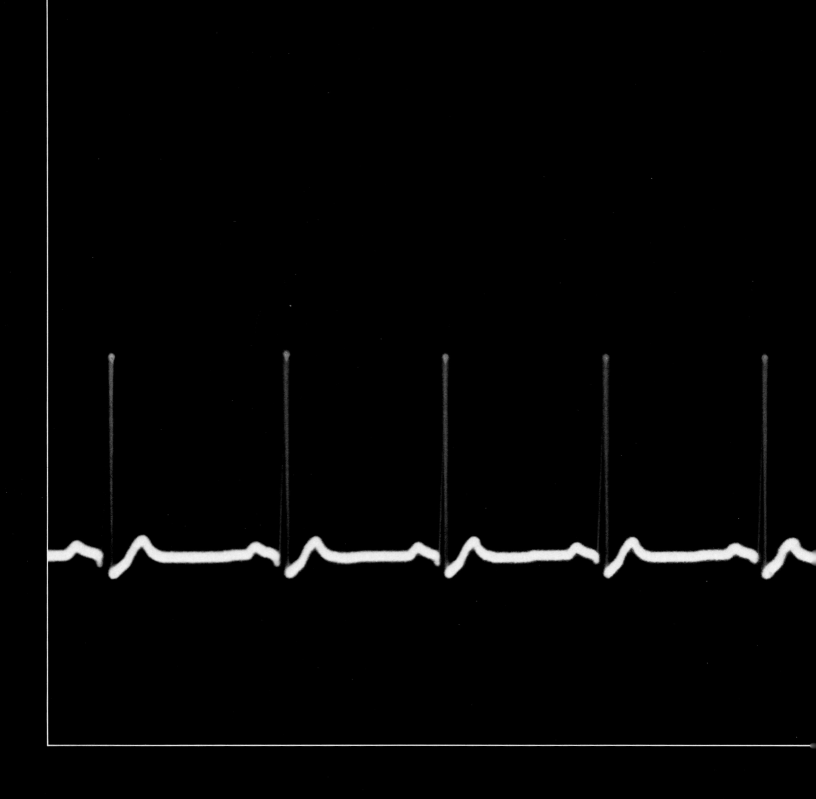

Monitoring Your Patient

Cardiac monitors

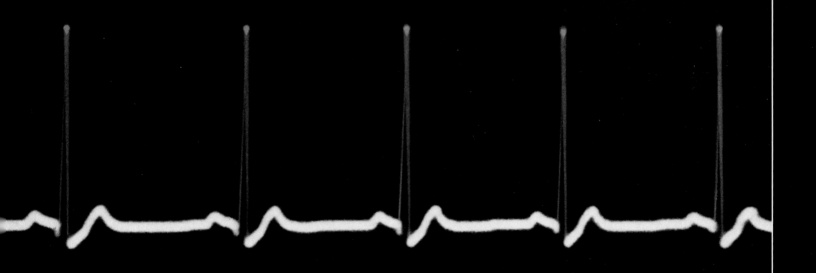

Cardiac monitors

You'll use a cardiac monitor when the doctor wants to learn about your patient's heart conduction. Do you know how a cardiac monitor works? Although the equipment and procedures are different, the principles of cardiac monitoring and electrocardiography are the same. Electrodes, applied to the patient, pick up the electrical impulses generated by his heart and send them to the monitor. Then, the monitor translates these impulses into a waveform that you or another health-care professional can analyze. In this way, you interpret your patient's cardiac condition.

Unlike electrocardiography, however, continuous cardiac monitoring is designed with the patient's comfort in mind. Instead of applying metal electrodes to your patient's arms and legs, which restrict movement, you'll apply light and comfortable disposable electrodes to your patient's chest. Other differences will be outlined on the following pages. There, we'll examine two monitoring systems: hardwire (or continuous) monitoring for around-the-clock monitoring of the patient on bed rest, and telemetry monitoring for around-the-clock monitoring of the convalescing patient. On page 128, we'll also examine a third type of cardiac monitoring: Holter monitoring, used on a 24-hour basis with patients undergoing cardiac rehabilitation.

Understanding monitors

Not all monitors are exactly alike, but every monitor features most of the components shown here. If your monitor's instrumentation panel differs significantly from this one, consult your operator's manual, supplied by the manufacturer.

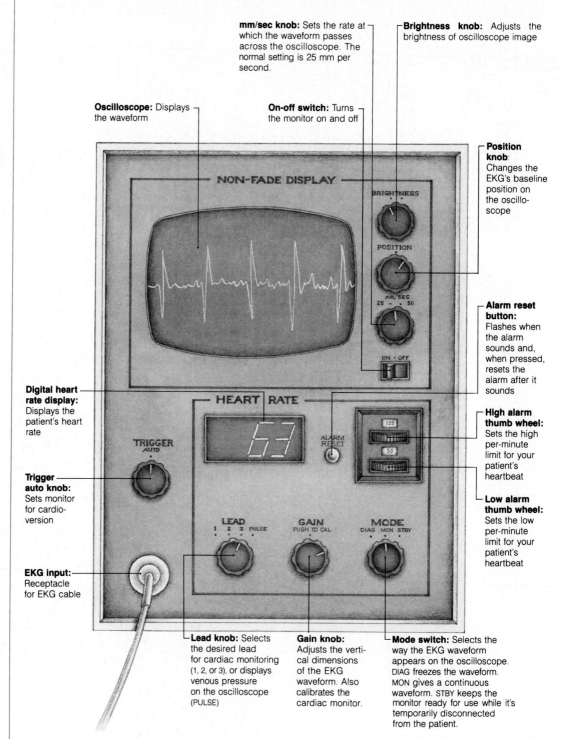

mm/sec knob: Sets the rate at which the waveform passes across the oscilloscope. The normal setting is 25 mm per second.

Brightness knob: Adjusts the brightness of oscilloscope image

Oscilloscope: Displays the waveform

On-off switch: Turns the monitor on and off

Position knob: Changes the EKG's baseline position on the oscilloscope

Alarm reset button: Flashes when the alarm sounds and, when pressed, resets the alarm after it sounds

Digital heart rate display: Displays the patient's heart rate

High alarm thumb wheel: Sets the high per-minute limit for your patient's heartbeat

Trigger auto knob: Sets monitor for cardioversion

Low alarm thumb wheel: Sets the low per-minute limit for your patient's heartbeat

EKG input: Receptacle for EKG cable

Lead knob: Selects the desired lead for cardiac monitoring (1, 2, or 3), or displays venous pressure on the oscilloscope (PULSE)

Gain knob: Adjusts the vertical dimensions of the EKG waveform. Also calibrates the cardiac monitor.

Mode switch: Selects the way the EKG waveform appears on the oscilloscope. DIAG freezes the waveform. MON gives a continuous waveform. STBY keeps the monitor ready for use while it's temporarily disconnected from the patient.

How to apply disposable electrodes

1 *Whichever type of continuous cardiac monitoring system you use, each employs disposable electrodes. You won't find it difficult to apply electrodes to your patient's skin, but you must do it correctly or you'll distort his EKG readings.*

Begin the procedure by assembling this equipment: three disposable floating electrodes, an alcohol swab, a safety razor with blade, and a sterile gauze pad.

The floating electrode is the most common and widely used electrode. It comes with a prejellied cushion underneath the electrode plate, to protect the patient's skin from direct contact. You'll find that this electrode's easy to apply, can remain on the patient's skin for days, and can conduct electrical impulses without distortion.

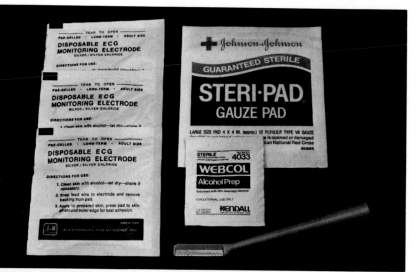

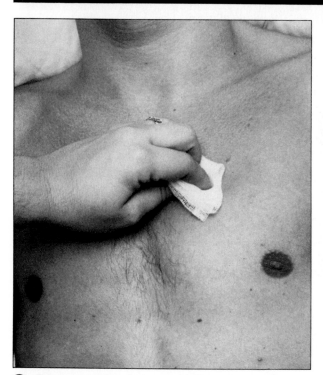

2 Tell your patient what you're going to do and why. Then, ask his permission to shave, if necessary, the small area on his chest where you'll apply the electrodes. Explain that the electrodes adhere better to skin that's been shaved. They also will be easier to remove.

Note: The sites you shave are determined by the doctor's lead choices. For more on leads and their placement, turn the page.

Prep the shaved area with an alcohol swab and let his skin dry completely. Then abrade his skin slightly with the gauze pad or some other rough material. Some floating electrodes are designed with a rough patch to rub on the skin.

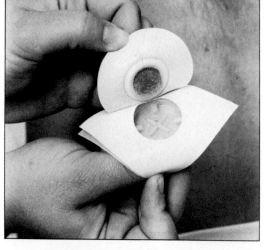

3 Peel off the paper backing on the electrode. As you do, avoid unnecessary contact with the adhesive ring. Check the sponge pad in the center of the electrode to see if it's moist with conductive jelly. If the sponge pad's dry, discard the electrode and open another one.

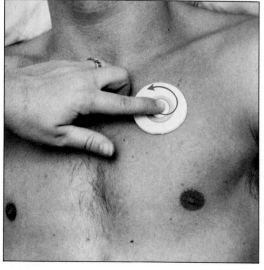

4 Place the electrode on the intended site with the adhesive side down. Then, ensure a good seal by applying pressure, beginning at the center of the electrode and moving outward. If you apply pressure by starting on one side and moving to the other, you could force out some of the conductive jelly from under the electrode, impairing conduction.

Follow the same procedure for applying the remaining electrodes.

Cardiac monitors

Nurses' guide to hardwire electrode placement

With five-electrode hardwire monitoring, as with a 12-lead EKG, you can record three standard limb leads (I, II, III), the three augmented limb leads (AVR, AVL, and AVF), and the six chest leads (V_1 through V_6) without distortion.

But, suppose you're using a monitor with only three electrodes. You can establish the three standard limb leads and the three augmented limb leads without difficulty, because each arrangement requires only three electrodes. But you can't establish the V_1 through V_6 chest leads because they require five electrodes. So, when you have a three-electrode monitor, use the modified chest leads described in this chart instead. These leads require only three electrodes, but yield readings similar to the V_1 and V_6 chest leads. Modified chest leads are abbreviated as MCL_1 and MCL_6. You'll find that for general monitoring on a three-electrode monitor, you'll probably use standard limb lead II, MCL_1, and MCL_6.

Type	Lead	Electrode placement	
Three-electrode monitor	Lead II	Positive (+): left side of chest, lowest palpable rib, midclavicular Negative (−): right shoulder, below clavicular hollow Ground (G): left shoulder, below clavicular hollow	
	MCL_1	Positive (+): right sternal border, lowest palpable rib Negative (−): left shoulder, below clavicular hollow Ground (G): right shoulder, below clavicular hollow	
	MCL_6	Positive (+): left side of chest, lowest palpable rib, midclavicular Negative (−): left shoulder, below clavicular hollow Ground (G): right shoulder, below clavicular hollow	
Five-electrode monitor	V_1 through V_6	Positive (+): left side of chest, just below lowest palpable rib Negative (−): right shoulder, midclavicular Ground (G): right side of chest, just below lowest palpable rib Inactive (I): left shoulder, midclavicular Chest V_1: fourth intercostal space to right of sternum Chest V_2: fourth intercostal space to left of sternum Chest V_3: halfway between V_2 and V_4 Chest V_4: fifth intercostal space, midclavicular, left side Chest V_5: halfway between V_4 and V_6 Chest V_6: fifth intercostal space at midaxillary line	

Initiating hardwire monitoring

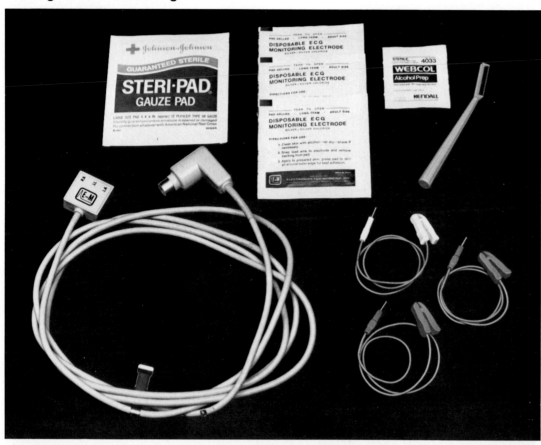

1 *Your patient is 75-year-old Violet Penski, who's suffered a myocardial infarction. Her doctor has ordered hardwire monitoring for her and it's your responsibility to initiate it. Do you know how? This photostory will show you, using a three-electrode monitor.*

Begin by gathering this equipment: three disposable floating electrodes, an alcohol swab, a sterile 4"x4" gauze pad, three lead wires, a lead wire receptacle and cable, and a razor, if needed. If your CCU is like most others, a cardiac monitor is permanently installed at your patient's bedside.

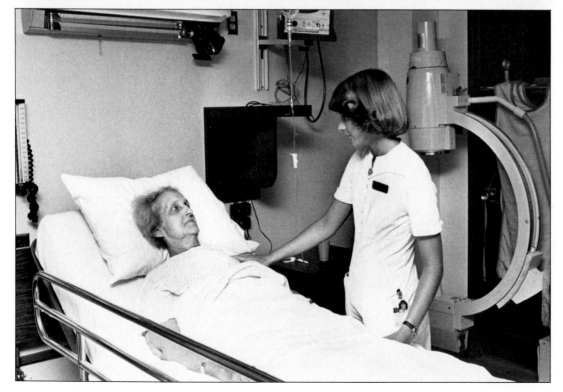

2 Explain the procedure to Mrs. Penski. Make sure you answer all her questions before proceeding.

Cardiac monitors

Initiating hardwire monitoring continued

3 The doctor has chosen lead II for monitoring Mrs. Penski. The chart on page 74 shows you where to apply the electrodes for that lead. After you apply them—using the procedure detailed on page 73—attach the lead wires to the three electrodes, as shown in the photo below.

How can you tell which lead wires attach to which electrodes? If your lead wires are marked +, −, G (and R if you're using a three-electrode telemetry monitor), attach them to their corresponding electrodes, as labeled in the chart on page 74.

But, what if your lead wires are coded RA, LA, LL, and, with five-electrode monitors, RL? Then, mentally divide your patient's chest into quadrants. Attach the RA lead wire to the electrode positioned nearest to the patient's right arm. Attach the RL lead wire to the electrode nearest to the patient's right leg, and so on. (The fifth lead wire of the five-electrode monitor attaches to the V or C electrode on the patient's chest.)

If your lead wires are color coded, consult the cardiac monitor operator's manual for instructions.

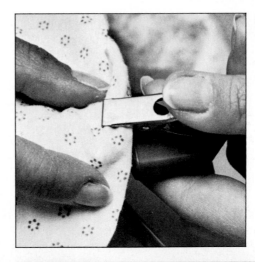

5 Fasten the lead wire receptacle to the patient's gown. This prevents undue stress on the lead wires when the patient moves.

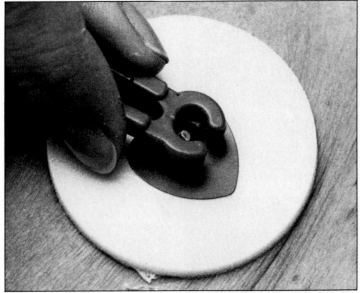

4 Attach the other ends of the lead wires to the lead wire receptacle. How can you tell which lead wires attach to which electrode outlets? The electrode outlets will be marked either with +, −, G symbols; RA, LA, RL abbreviations; or colors. Know your system's markings.

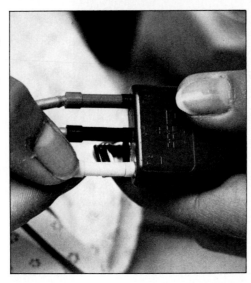

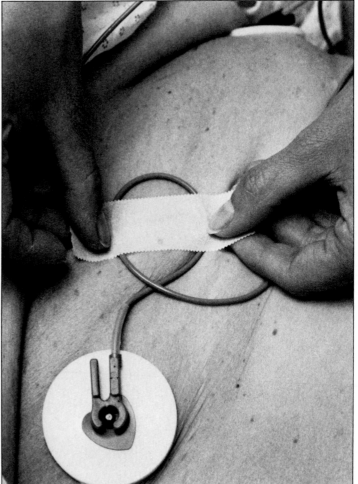

6 Form a stress loop in each lead wire, and tape it to the patient's skin, as shown here. Leave enough slack between the electrodes and the stress loop to allow for patient movement without straining the electrode connection.

Important: Is your patient allergic to adhesive tape? Use non-allergenic tape instead.

7 Plug the lead wire receptacle cable into the bedside monitor.

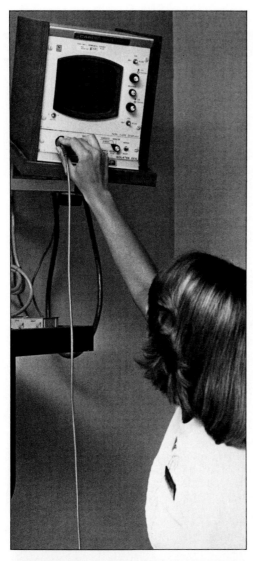

9 How tall is the QRS complex you're getting? It must be tall enough for the monitor to record each beat. But don't make it so tall that it barely fits on the oscilloscope screen.

If you want to enlarge the QRS complex, set the GAIN switch to 2. If you want to decrease it, set the GAIN switch to 1.

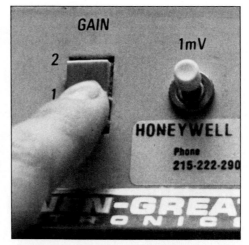

10 Next, calibrate the monitor by pressing the button marked 1mv or CAL, (depending on the manufacturer of the equipment). This will produce a 1 millivolt high waveform on the oscilloscope. If the R wave of the QRS complex isn't higher than the 1 millivolt waveform, adjust the GAIN setting so it is.

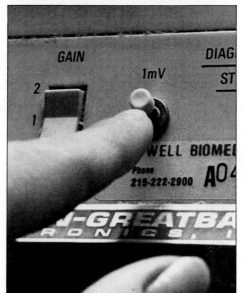

8 Turn the HOLD-RUN-RECORD switch to RUN.

Then, turn the mode switch from STANDBY to MONITOR. Expect a tracing to appear in about 20 seconds.

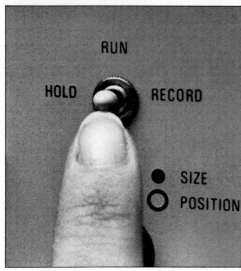

11 Then, if necessary, turn the position knob to center the waveform on the oscilloscope.

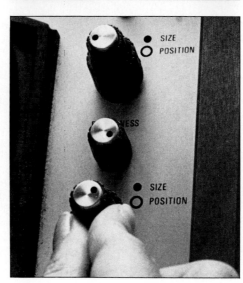

Cardiac monitors

Initiating hardwire monitoring continued

12 Your monitoring system either has a central console, or a self-contained bedside monitor. If your hospital uses a central console, find the group of controls on the console face that corresponds to the controls on the bedside monitor. Touch only these controls. If you're using a self-contained bedside monitor, continue the procedure there.

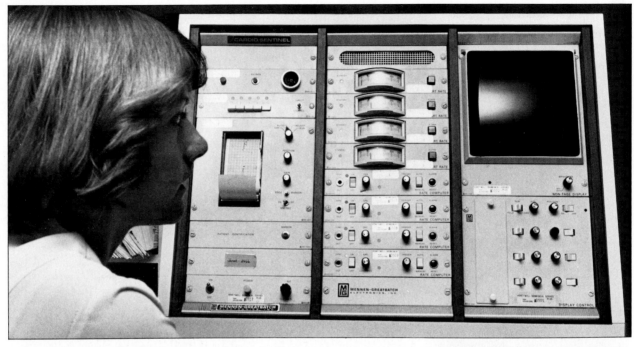

13 Set the HIGH alarm at 120 beats per minute and the LOW alarm at 50 beats per minute, unless the doctor orders otherwise.

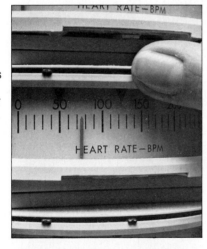

14 Set the heart rate alarm to AUTO, so it'll sound whenever the patient's heart rate goes above or below the limits you've set.

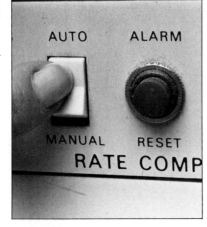

15 Now, check to see if each QRS complex on the oscilloscope is being counted by the monitor. First, turn on the audible QRS signal. It will sound with each QRS complex counted. You can also tell if they're counted by watching the rate light. If the audible alarm doesn't sound, or the rate light doesn't blink with each complex, increase the GAIN setting until the QRS complex is of sufficient height to trigger these signals every time.

Note: If you're working at a central console, don't make the QRS complex so tall that it interferes with other waveforms on the console's oscilloscope. Adjust the size and position of the waveform as you did on the bedside monitor.

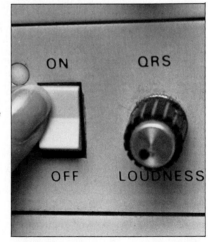

16 Turn the recorder to AUTO and the SWEEP to 25 mm/sec. With these settings, if the patient's heart rate sets off the alarm, the recorder will print as fast as the oscilloscope reading.

Finally, check the paper in the recorder. If a refill is needed, add more paper, following the instructions in the operator's manual.

Now you've initiated hardwire monitoring. It will give you a continuous record of Mrs. Penski's heartbeat during her hospitalization.

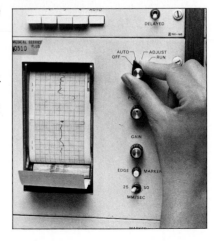

Caring for the patient being monitored

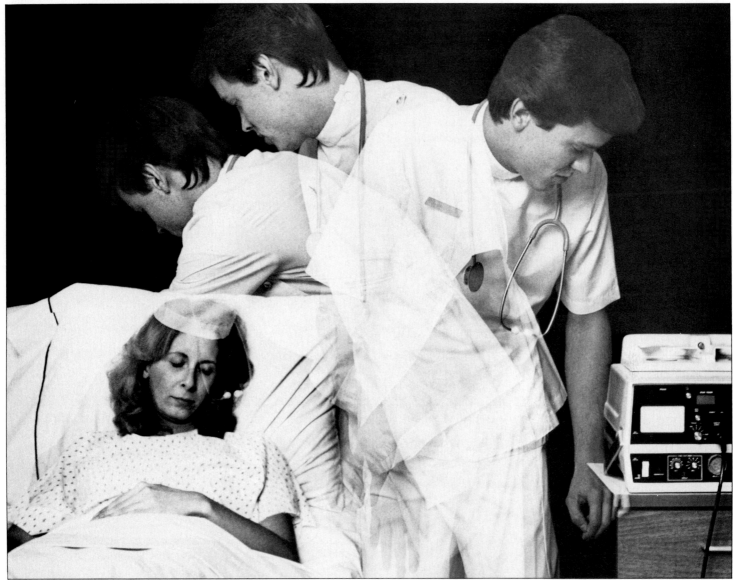

Patient care is a difficult skill to master. It requires a great deal of time, perseverance, empathy, and energy—things in constant demand in all hospitals. But when a patient is on a cardiac monitor, the requirements are even greater. You must set up and maintain sophisticated equipment, without forgetting or ignoring your patient. Here are some guidelines to help you meet her physical—and emotional—needs:

Explain the monitoring procedure to her step by step, so she knows what to expect. Tell her why she's being monitored and how it helps. Investigate what she knows about monitoring, then clear up any misconceptions. For example, is she afraid the alarm will go off when she moves? Does she think she'll get a shock from the electrodes? Anticipate such concerns and try to relieve her anxieties. Sound the alarm so she knows what to expect. Tell her that false alarms are a likely occurrence and shouldn't upset her.

Finally, make sure the monitor doesn't face the patient. For one not familiar with cardiac waveforms, your patient may become unnecessarily agitated watching EKG waveform fluctuations.

During monitoring, don't place more importance on the monitor than on your patient. *When you enter her room, greet her first and attend to her needs before you go to the monitor.* Don't discuss her condition with others at her bedside unless you include her in the discussions, too. If the monitor sounds an alarm, fight your natural inclination to look toward the source of the sound: the monitor. Even if you suspect that the monitor's malfunctioning—and the alarm's not an indication that the patient's condition is deteriorating—don't take any chances. First, determine without question that your patient doesn't need attention. Then, look at the equipment. This method not only safeguards your patient's health, but it eliminates time-wasting guesswork by drawing attention to the most likely problems first.

Keep in mind that a cardiac monitor is only a *tool* of nursing. It doesn't replace the attention and care you can give a patient, and never will. Your keen observations are the best monitor of your patient's well-being.

Cardiac monitors

Learning about telemetry monitoring

Have you ever used telemetry monitoring? If you have, then you know it requires three basic pieces of equipment: a transmitter with electrodes, relay wires (usually recessed in the hospital ceiling), and a central console. You'll use the electrodes to attach the transmitter to your patient's body. Telemetry monitoring doesn't restrict the patient's movement as much as hardwire monitoring does. But telemetry's still somewhat limiting, because its relay wires can pick up the patient's heartbeat only within a certain distance from the central console. That distance, ranging from 50 to 2,000 feet (15 to 610 m), depends on the make of your equipment and your unit's floor plan.

To learn more about telemetry monitoring, read on.

Nurses' guide to telemetry electrode placement

The telemetry system your hospital uses features either two or three electrodes. As this chart shows, both types can monitor in the standard lead II position or the MCL_1 position. But the three-electrode type also allows you to monitor in the MCL_6 position.

Note the reference electrode in the three-electrode monitor leads. The reference electrode is designed to reduce distortion and amplify the transmitted EKG signal, but most two-electrode monitors do this effectively without it.

Type	Lead	Electrode placement
Two-electrode monitor	Lead II 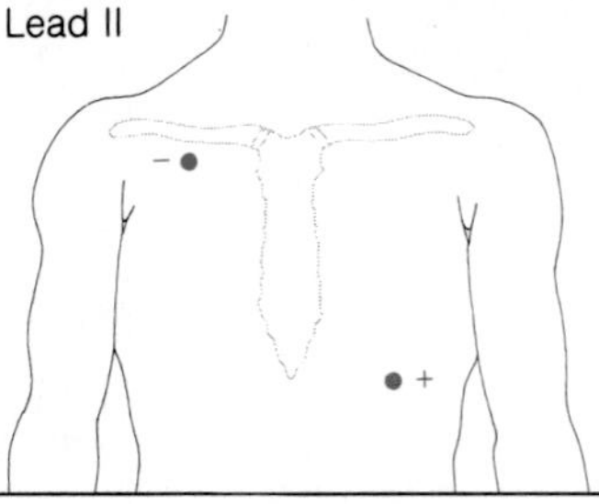	Positive (+): left side of chest, lowest palpable rib, midclavicular Negative (−): right shoulder, below clavicular hollow Ground (G): not applied to patient (built into console)
	MCL_1 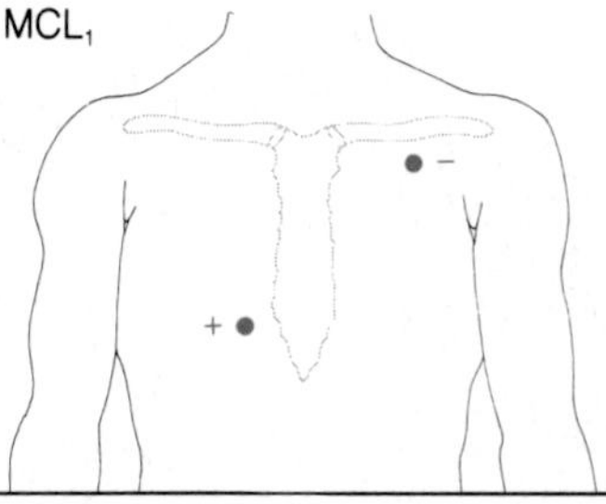	Positive (+): right sternal border, lowest palpable rib Negative (−): left shoulder, below clavicular hollow Ground (G): not applied to patient (built into console)
Three-electrode monitor	Lead II 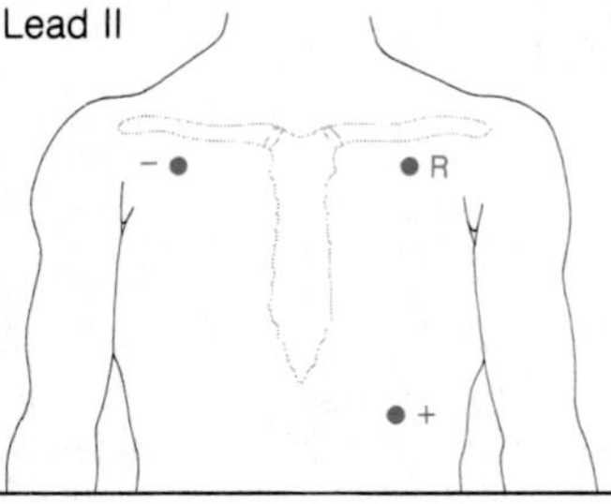	Positive (+): left side of chest, lowest palpable rib, midclavicular Negative (−): right shoulder, below clavicular hollow Ground (G): not applied to patient, built into console Reference (R): left shoulder, below clavicular hollow
	MCL_1 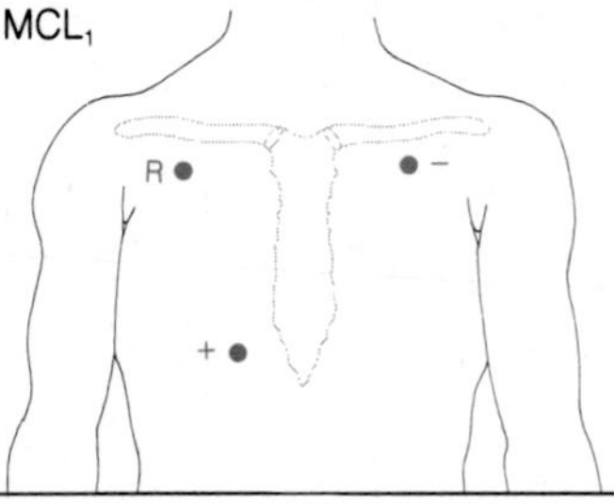	Positive (+): right sternal border, lowest palpable rib Negative (−): left shoulder, below clavicular hollow Ground (G): not applied to patient (built into console) Reference (R): right shoulder, below clavicular hollow
	MCL_6 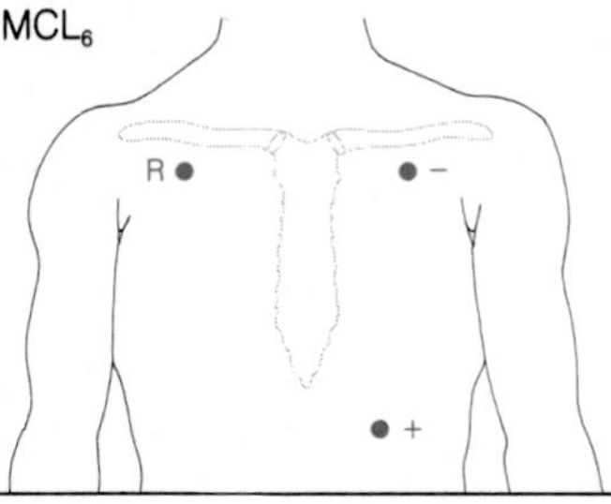	Positive (+): left side, lowest palpable rib, midclavicular Negative (−): left shoulder, below clavicular hollow Ground (G): not applied to patient (built into console) Reference (R): right shoulder, below clavicular hollow

Initiating telemetry monitoring

1 *Hans Wilheim, a 48-year-old house painter, is recovering from an anterior wall myocardial infarction. He's been transferred to your unit for telemetry monitoring. Do you know how to set up such a monitor? If not, this photostory will show you.*

Begin by gathering the equipment shown in the inset to use with the telemetry console: a telemetry transmitter, two or three electrodes (depending on the transmitter), a transmitter pouch, and a battery.

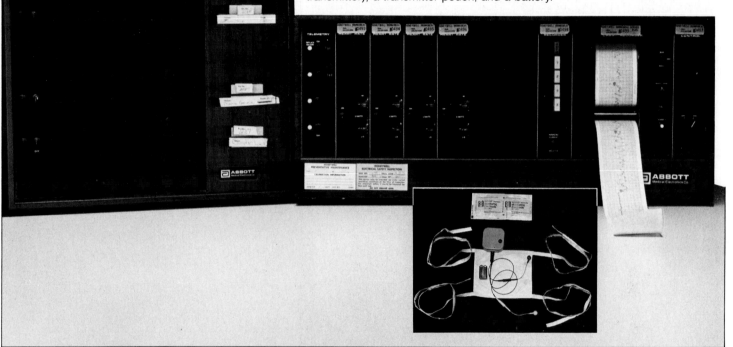

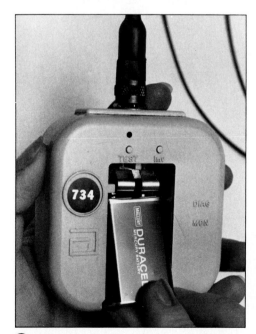

2 Insert the battery into the transmitter. Make sure you match the polarity markings on the battery with those on the transmitter case.

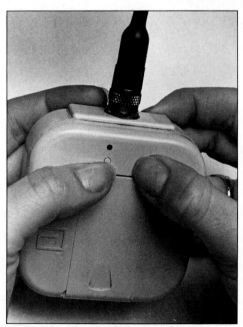

3 Then, test the battery by pushing the tiny test light button on the back of the transmitter. If that doesn't cause the test light to go on, get a new battery.

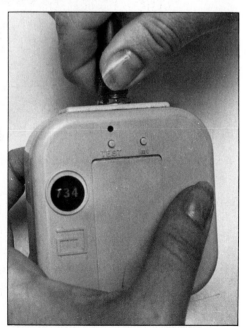

4 Make sure the lead wire cable's securely attached to the transmitter.

Now you're ready to explain the procedure to the patient.

Cardiac monitors

Initiating telemetry monitoring continued

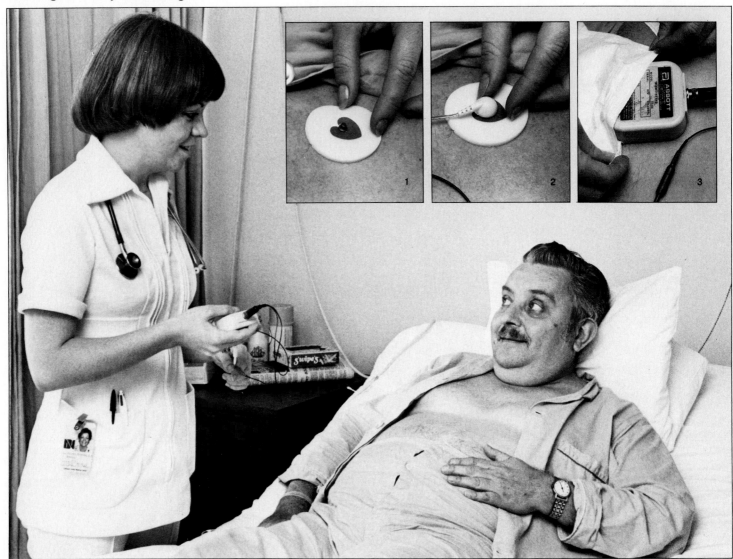

5 Show the transmitter to the patient and explain how it works, as the nurse is doing in the photo above. Before proceeding, answer any questions he has.

[Inset 1] Apply the electrodes to his chest, using the procedure explained on page 73. Arrange them to establish the lead ordered by the doctor.

[Inset 2] Attach lead wires to the electrodes, following the pattern outlined in step 3 on page 76.

[Inset 3] Now, place the transmitter into a carrying pouch. Telemetry manufacturers usually supply cotton pouches with their transmitters, but your hospital may use handmade ones.

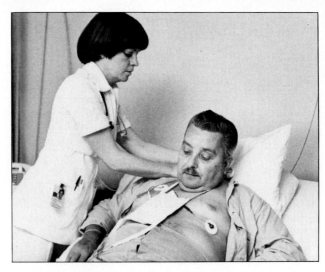

6 Tie the pouch strings around your patient's neck and torso. Make sure the pouch is secure, but take care that your patient's not uncomfortable.

7 Now, go to the monitor's central console. On the front panel, find the group of controls with the number that corresponds to the number of the telemetry transmitter you've just connected. Activate the transmitter by turning the switch to ON.

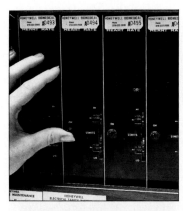

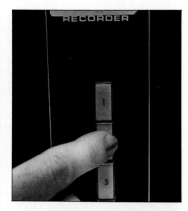

9 Now, turn on the RECORDER button. A waveform printout will begin immediately.

8 Set the HIGH alarm and LOW alarm limits, at rates the doctor orders. But first, test the alarms by setting the limits well within the patient's normal rate. When they sound, turn them off, and adjust them as ordered. *Note:* Some telemetry monitors also have an ALARM button, in addition to the high and low settings. If the monitor you're using does, press the ALARM button to make sure it's working, too.

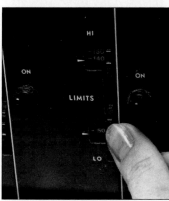

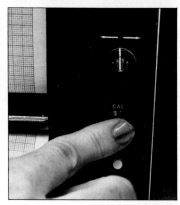

10 Push the CAL button to get a 1 millivolt high waveform. If the QRS complex is less than 1 millivolt, turn the GAIN CONTROL knob until the complex exceeds 1 millivolt. Now, the monitor is assured of picking up each heartbeat.

Turn the recorder button to AUTO so the recorder will automatically begin a printout of the heartbeat if the alarm sounds. Now, you've initiated telemetry monitoring.

Troubleshooting cardiac monitors

This chart shows you how to troubleshoot the common problems you're apt to encounter while working with a cardiac monitor. Consider this a supplement to the cardiography troubleshooting chart on page 49. As you study both charts, keep in mind that no matter what problem arises with the equipment—from a straight line on the oscilloscope to a sparking monitor—always examine your patient first.

Problem	Possible causes	Solution
Skin excoriation under electrode	• Patient allergic to electrode adhesive • Electrode left on skin too long	• Remove electrodes and apply nonallergenic electrodes and nonallergenic tape. • Remove electrode, clean site, and reapply electrode at new site.
Broken lead wires or broken cable	• Not using stress loops on lead wires • Cleaning cables and lead wires with alcohol or acetone, causing brittleness	• Replace lead wires and retape them, using stress loops. • Clean cable and lead wires with soapy water instead of alcohol or acetone. *Important:* Do not get cable ends wet.
Double-triggering (P wave and QRS complex, or QRS complex and T wave are of equal height)	• Monitor GAIN setting too high, particularly with MCL$_1$ setting	• Reset GAIN setting. If possible, monitor patient on MCL$_6$ or another available lead.
Alarm sounds, but you see no evidence of arrhythmia	• QRS complex too small to register • QRS complex not registering because of MCL$_1$ lead setting • HIGH alarm set too low, or LOW alarm set too high • Artifact (waveform interference)	• Reapply electrodes. • Set GAIN so that the height of the complex is greater than 1 millivolt. • If possible, monitor the patient on MCL$_6$. • Set alarm limits according to patient's heart rate. • Check electrodes and reapply them, if necessary.

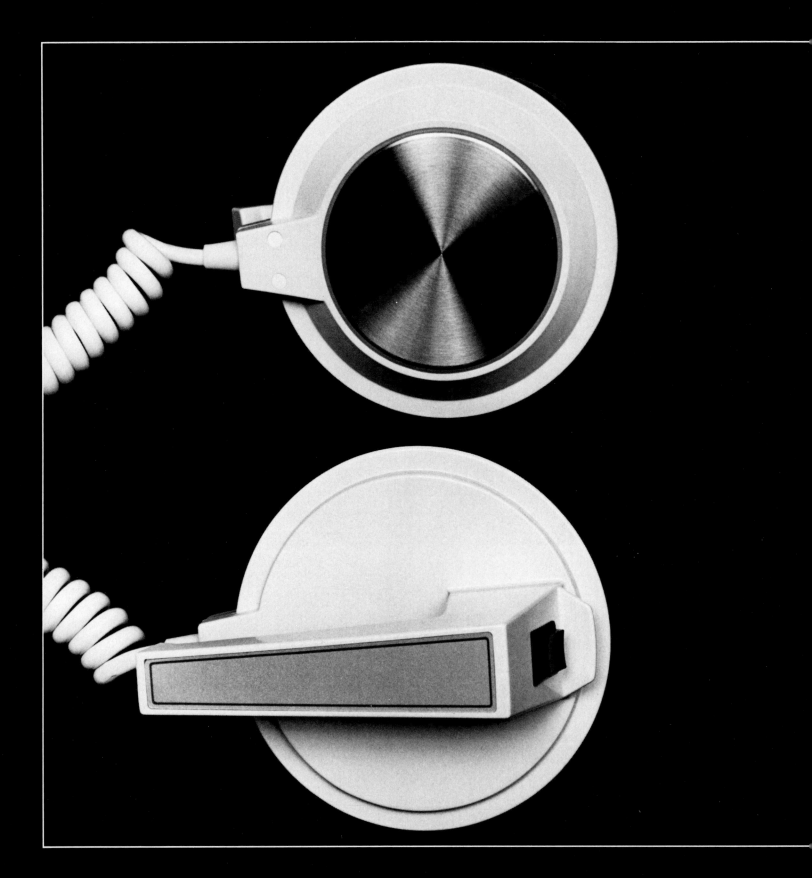

Dealing with Cardiac Complications

Emergency procedures

Cardiac pacemakers

Emergency procedures

Cardiac emergency! It can happen to a person on the street or to a patient in the most sophisticated CCU. In either case, your response could mean the difference between life and death. That's why, regardless of where you work, you've been trained in cardiopulmonary resuscitation. But you should also be familiar with these lifesaving procedures:
- defibrillating your patient
- performing cardioversion
- applying rotating tourniquets
- helping to insert an intra-aortic balloon.

You can find out about these procedures and more by reading the following pages.

Learning about cardiac failure

Cardiac failure means the heart [...] enough blood through the body [...] ordinary demands. To understan[...] happens during cardiac failure, [...] some basic anatomy. The heart [...] of two separate, but related, pum[...] tems: the heart's left side, or the s[...] circulation pump, and the heart's [...] or the pulmonary circulation pum[...] failure does not necessarily involv[...] sides of the heart. Certain physic[...] may alter the functioning of one [...] without initially impairing the oth[...]

Because the heart's left side c[...] involved work, it is taxed more th[...] heart's right side and is more like[...] into failure than that side. While [...] heart failure may occur first in th[...] of right ventricular infarction or p[...] hypertension, it usually occurs a[...] as a result of left-sided heart fail[...] you treat left-sided heart failure [...] and successfully, you can avoid [...] heart failure.

Performing cardiopulmonary resuscitation (CPR)

1 *As a nurse, you may be called on to perform cardiopulmonary resuscitation (CPR) more often than any other emergency procedure. That's why, no matter where you work, you should be trained in CPR by a certified instructor. If you haven't performed CPR in a while, use this photostory to refresh your memory.*

You're caring for a patient in the CCU. His cardiac monitor alarm sounds and the waveform on the oscilloscope tells you he's suffering cardiac arrest (see inset). What do you do? First, assess his condition by checking for a carotid pulse. If you feel nothing, give him a precordial thump. This must be done within 1 minute of a monitored cardiac arrest and shouldn't be attempted under any other circumstances.

Here's how to do it: Using the fleshy portion of your fist, deliver a sharp blow to the patient's midsternum. Immediately check the cardiac monitor for signs of a restored heartbeat. To double-check, feel the patient's

2 Make sure your patient's lying on a firm surface. If he's on a bed or a stretcher, put a board under him.

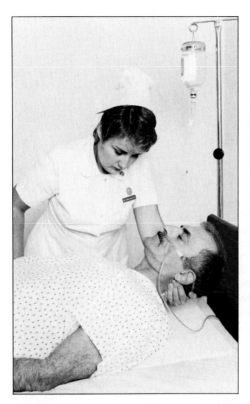

3 Open the patient's airway by hyperextending his neck. Then, ventilate his lungs with four quick, full breaths before you proceed further.

If you haven't already done so, pull down the patient's gown to expose his chest.

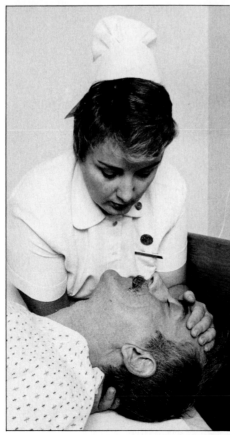

4 Now, position yourself for chest compressions by kneeling or standing beside the patient. If your patient is on a stretcher, stand on a stool.

Here's how to position your hands. Begin by locating the xiphoid process, which is at the lower end of the patient's sternum. Measure 1½″ to 2″ (4 to 5 cm)—or approximately two finger widths— up from this point. You'll give chest compressions here.

Important: Never give chest compressions directly over the patient's xiphoid process or you'll lacerate his liver.

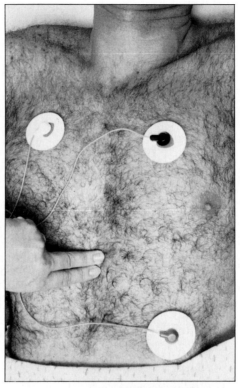

5 Now, place one hand on top of the other, as the nurse is doing here. Interlock your fingers so you're sure of keeping them off the patient's chest wall.

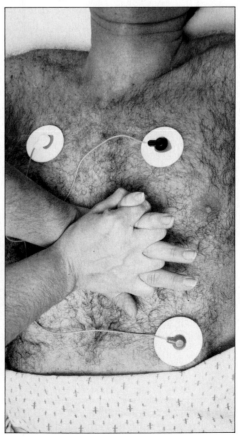

Emergency procedures

Performing cardiopulmonary resuscitation (CPR) continued

6 As the nurse is beginning to do here, lean forward so that your shoulders are directly over the patient's sternum and your arms are at a 90° angle to his chest (see arrow). Keep your arms straight to minimize fatigue and to use your weight effectively.

With the heel of your hand, exert pressure downward, depressing the patient's sternum 1½" to 2" (4 to 5 cm). This action squeezes the heart between the sternum and vertebral column and forces blood from the heart's chambers.

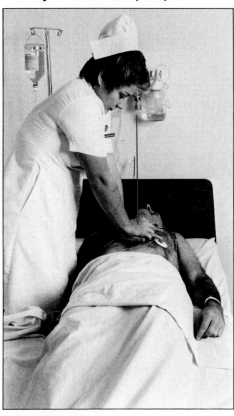

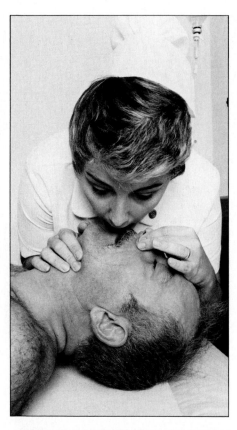

8 Then, deliver two quick lung inflations. Deliver these breaths in rapid succession, without allowing the patient to exhale fully between breaths. Then, resume chest compressions.

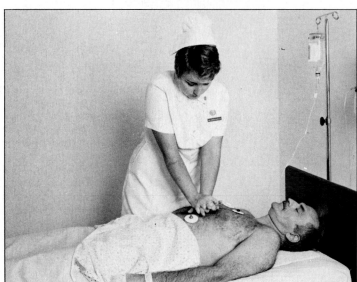

7 After each chest compression, release all pressure. This allows the sternum to return to its normal position, and permits the heart's chambers to refill.

Important: Don't remove your hands from the patient's chest when you release pressure on his sternum. Doing so may cause you to lose correct hand placement.

Work smoothly and rhythmically, making sure compression and relaxation times are equal. To maintain this rhythm, count aloud, "One, and two, and three, and four," up to fifteen.

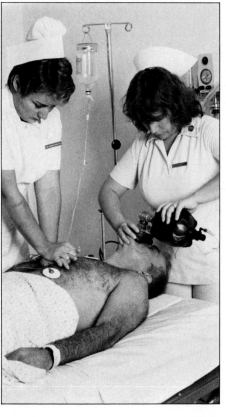

9 If you're in a CCU, someone probably will have arrived by this time with an AMBU™ hand-held resuscitator. The assisting nurse will remove the bed's headboard (for better positioning) and continue inflating the patient's lungs while you apply chest compressions.

For two-person CPR, give one lung inflation after every five chest compressions. Count aloud, "One-one thousand, two-one thousand, three-one thousand, four one-thousand, five one-thousand."

Then, the assisting nurse should deliver a lung inflation quickly, so there's no pause in chest compressions.

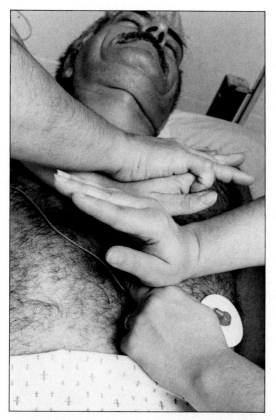

10 If you get tired and need to switch positions with the assisting nurse, notify her by saying (in rhythm), "Switch-two-three-four-breathe." On the word "breathe," the assisting nurse should deliver one quick inflation, move over to the patient's chest, and locate the xiphoid process. Then, with her opposite hand, she should push your hands away (replacing them with her own). Without interrupting the established rhythm, she resumes the count.

Important: When you're doing two-person CPR, never remove your hands from the patient's chest until your helper pushes them away.

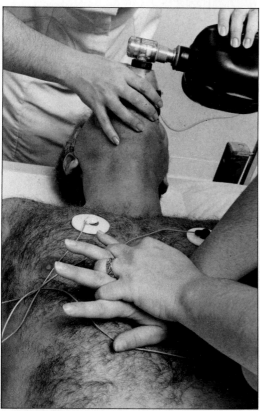

11 Move immediately to the patient's head and check for possible pulse. If there is no pulse, deliver a lung inflation at the count of five.

For information on how to give CPR to an infant or a child, see the NURSING PHOTOBOOK *Dealing with Emergencies.*

Treating cardiac disorders with drugs

If your patient has cardiac failure or cardiac arrhythmias, one of the doctor's first steps will be to initiate drug therapy. He has a good reason for this. Drugs are a relatively simple, effective way to deal with cardiac abnormalities.

Before we can understand how drugs affect the heart, let's review some cardiac physiology. The myocardium, or cardiac muscle, contracts and relaxes because of a chemical ion exchange that occurs in every myocardial cell. As the cell exchanges its normal ion makeup for ions surrounding it (depolarization), its action potential or level of electrical activity peaks. Then, as the cell returns to its normal chemical makeup, (repolarization), its action potential decreases.

Automaticity describes the ability of certain myocardial cells to depolarize spontaneously. These cells make up the heart's sinoatrial (SA) node and surrounding tissue, the atrioventricular (AV) junction, the bundle of His, and the Purkinje fiber tissues. Cardiac problems occur when the AV junction, bundle of His, or Purkinje fibers depolarize at a faster rate than the SA node.

Timing, or electrical conduction velocity, is also important. If the impulse conduction of the SA node is slowed or suppressed, the AV junction generates its own impulse to replace the slowed or lost one. If conduction velocity is altered, depolarization will become random, causing arrhythmias.

Relative and functional refractory periods refer to those times when the depolarization/repolarization process can be altered. However, when the myocardial cell's action potential peaks, the cell resists restimulation or change. This is called the absolute refractory period. As the action potential decreases, the cell becomes more and more receptive to restimulation.

Different drugs affect automaticity, conduction, velocity, and refractory periods. Digitalis glycosides, for example, can help a patient with cardiac failure by making his heart work more efficiently. It alters the heart's automaticity, conduction velocity, and refractory periods, resulting in increased contractility—greater pumping action—which restores proper atrial perfusion.

If the patient has a ventricular arrhythmia, the doctor may order an antiarrhythmic drug, such as quinidine. This drug depresses the heart's automaticity and prolongs the relative and functional refractory period. As a result, ventricular arrhythmias are suppressed.

For more information about effects of specific drugs on the heart, see page 144.

Emergency procedures

Learning about countershock therapy

As you know, countershock therapy (defibrillation and cardioversion) involves delivering a high-intensity electrical charge to the heart. The charge's purpose is to depolarize the myocardium, stopping the heart's abnormal electrical activity and clearing the way for the sinoatrial (SA) node to assume conduction control. If all works well, this restores a cardiac rhythm. The doctor may order countershock therapy after trying drug treatment, or if the arrhythmia has become life threatening.

Defibrillation delivers a *random electrical shock* to the heart. You'll use this type of countershock therapy primarily to treat ventricular fibrillation and asystole.

Cardioversion delivers a *synchronized electrical shock* to the heart. The cardioverter delivers the shock in synchronization with the R wave of the patient's EKG. By using synchronization, you avoid shocking the heart in the vulnerable period of the relative refractory phase, which could cause ventricular fibrillation. When drug therapy has failed, or the arrhythmia's become life threatening, the doctor may choose cardioversion to treat ventricular tachycardia and abnormal atrial rhythms, such as atrial flutter and fibrillation.

Defibrillating your patient

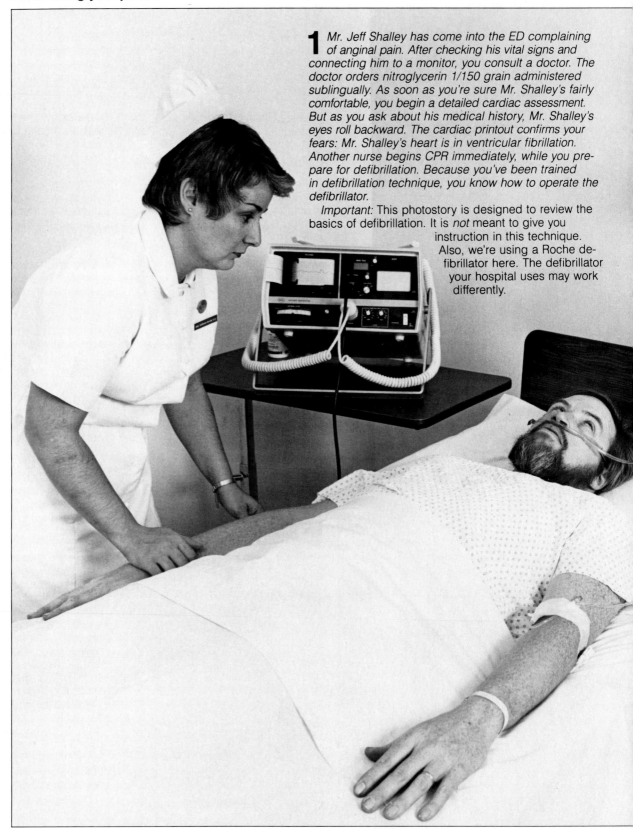

1 Mr. Jeff Shalley has come into the ED complaining of anginal pain. After checking his vital signs and connecting him to a monitor, you consult a doctor. The doctor orders nitroglycerin 1/150 grain administered sublingually. As soon as you're sure Mr. Shalley's fairly comfortable, you begin a detailed cardiac assessment. But as you ask about his medical history, Mr. Shalley's eyes roll backward. The cardiac printout confirms your fears: Mr. Shalley's heart is in ventricular fibrillation. Another nurse begins CPR immediately, while you prepare for defibrillation. Because you've been trained in defibrillation technique, you know how to operate the defibrillator.

Important: This photostory is designed to review the basics of defibrillation. It is *not* meant to give you instruction in this technique. Also, we're using a Roche defibrillator here. The defibrillator your hospital uses may work differently.

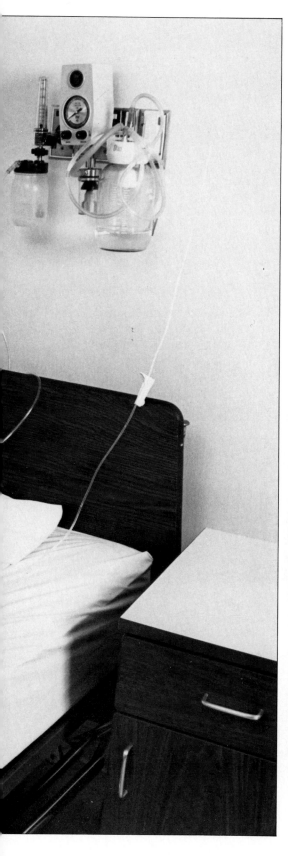

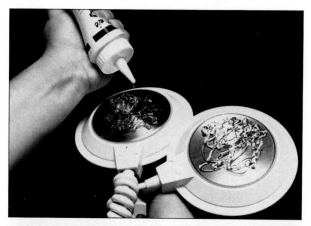

2 Begin by turning on the defibrillator. Then, squeeze generous amounts of conductive jelly onto each defibrillator paddle, as the nurse is doing here. The jelly conducts electricity and, at the same time, reduces the risk of electrical burns.

Nursing tip: Always keep a tube or bottle of conductive jelly with the defibrillator. If jelly's not available, place saline-soaked pads on your patient's chest instead. But don't use alcohol pads. They may ignite.

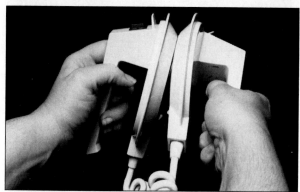

3 Coat the entire surface of each paddle with jelly by rubbing them together. Don't rub them so hard that jelly oozes onto the sides of the paddles or onto your hands. If that happens, remove the excess jelly with a cloth before proceeding.

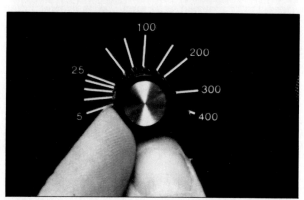

4 Following the doctor's orders, or your hospital's standard procedure, select the correct electrical charge on the defibrillator control panel. Chances are, the doctor's ordered 200 to 300 joules, the average charge for an adult.

Note: If your defibrillator measures the charge in watt-seconds instead of joules, set the charge at 200 to 300 watt-seconds, a comparable amount.

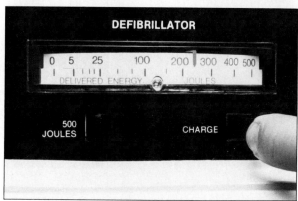

5 Press the charge button on the control panel to charge the paddles. When the display registers the electrical charge you selected, release the charge button.

Emergency procedures

Defibrillating your patient continued

6 As a precaution, look at the patient's EKG rhythm strip one more time to make sure he still needs defibrillation.

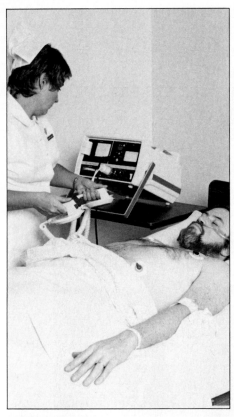

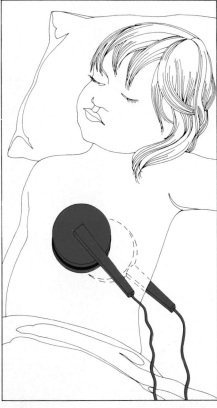

8 If the defibrillator paddles differ from the ones shown in this photostory, *or* if your patient is an infant or small child, position the paddles this way: place the posterior paddle on your patient's back, between his shoulder blades. Place the anterior paddle on his chest, between his left nipple and sternum.

In either case, make sure the paddles rest flat against the patient's skin. If they don't, you may cause a dangerous electrical arc, which can burn you and your patient. You can also cause electrical arcing by failing to keep the paddles at least 2″ (5 cm) apart at all times.

7 Then, place the paddles on the patient's chest, as shown here. Put one paddle to the right of his sternum between his second and third intercostal spaces, and the other at the fifth intercostal space, left midclavicular line, near the apex of the heart.

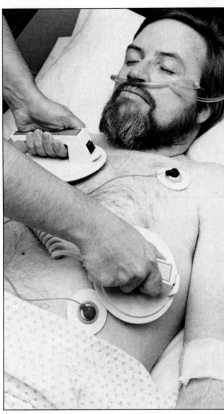

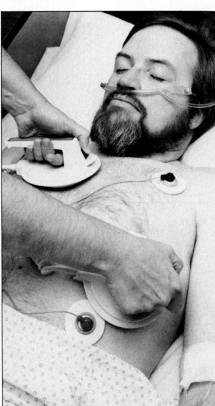

9 When you've positioned the paddles correctly, tell everyone to stand clear of the patient and his bed. If your patient's receiving oxygen, make sure it's turned off. Check to make sure you're not standing on a wet surface. Announce once more that everyone should step back. Then, to discharge the defibrillator, simultaneously press the red discharge buttons on both handles, as the nurse is doing here. This delivers an electrical shock to your patient's heart designed to halt his ventricular fibrillation.

10 Check the patient's EKG strip to see if you've altered his heart rhythm. If necessary, have a coworker resume CPR.

After delivering the shock, remove the paddles. Examine the patient's skin for burns. If any are present, make a mental note of their size and appearance, so you can document them in your nurses' notes after the procedure.

Then, on the EKG strip, record the date, time, lead, and prescribed electrical charge. After 1 minute, ask your coworker to stop CPR so you can check your patient's heart rhythm again. If defibrillation and CPR haven't produced the desired rhythm change, the doctor may want you to repeat defibrillation. Before you can do this, you must recharge the paddles (see step 5), maintaining CPR all the while.

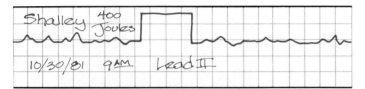

Shalley 400 Joules
10/30/81   9AM   Lead II

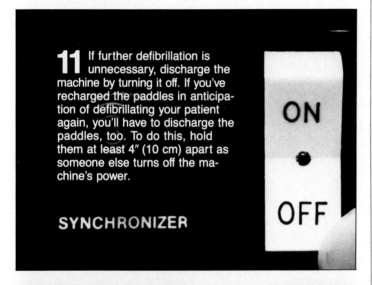

11 If further defibrillation is unnecessary, discharge the machine by turning it off. If you've recharged the paddles in anticipation of defibrillating your patient again, you'll have to discharge the paddles, too. To do this, hold them at least 4" (10 cm) apart as someone else turns off the machine's power.

SYNCHRONIZER

ON
OFF

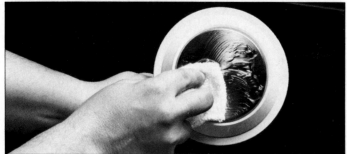

12 Once the machine's discharged, clean the paddles with soap and water, making sure you remove all conductive jelly. Any jelly that remains will corrode the metal paddle heads, which can cause electrical arcing and skin burns the next time the paddles are used.

To prepare the defibrillator for immediate reuse, make sure the lead selector is set properly, and the machine is stocked with conductive jelly or saline-soaked pads.

Testing the defibrillator

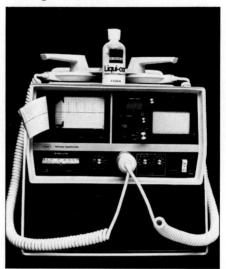

1 *Because defibrillation is an emergency procedure, you won't have time to gather and test the necessary equipment moments before you use it. Everything must be in its place ahead of time, including a supply of conductive jelly or saline-soaked pads. Here we'll show you how to test the Roche defibrillator. To test your hospital's defibrillator, read your operator's manual.*

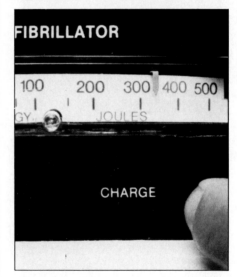

FIBRILLATOR

100   200   300   400   500
JOULES

CHARGE

2 Someone in your unit should be responsible for testing the defibrillator daily. To do this, she should follow this procedure: Set the defibrillator at 300 joules. Depress the charge button on the defibrillator until the display number matches the joules setting.

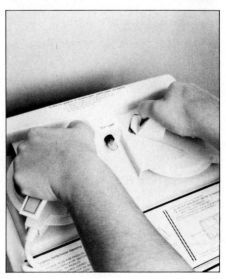

3 Leave the paddles in their resting place on the defibrillator as you simultaneously push the red discharge buttons on both handles.

If the paddles deliver the correct electrical charge (300 joules), the test light will flash on. Use the defibrillator with confidence.

If the test light doesn't flash on, get the defibrillator repaired as soon as possible.

Emergency procedures

Performing cardioversion

1 *Forty-seven-year-old Carl Reilly has rapid atrial flutter that hasn't responded to antiarrhythmic drug therapy. Because his arrhythmia is overworking his heart and causing decreased cardiac output, the doctor decides to perform cardioversion.*

Gather this equipment: synchronized defibrillator (with built-in cardiac monitor), conductive jelly, a hand-held resuscitator, (such as this Airshields AMBU™ Bag), a blood-pressure cuff, and a stethoscope.

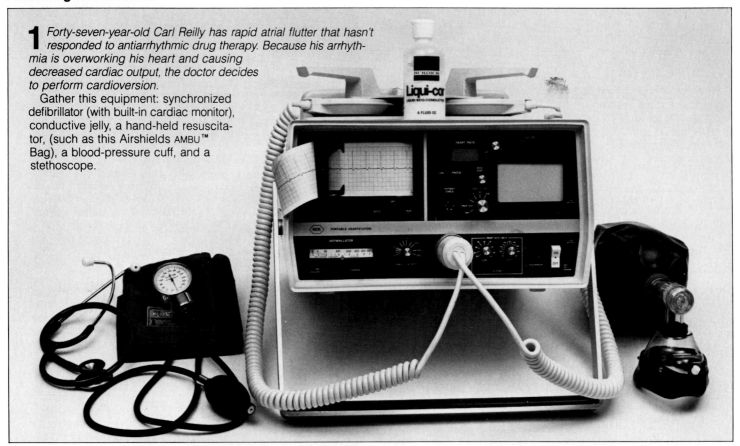

2 Begin the procedure by reinforcing what the doctor told the patient he was going to do and why. Don't use the word *shock* in your explanation. Tell him instead that cardioversion uses electrical current to slow down his heart rate and relieve some of his symptoms. Answer all his questions. Then, since cardioversion's elective therapy, make sure the patient has signed a consent form.

Then, establish baseline vital signs by taking your patient's blood pressure, temperature, pulse rate, and respiration rate. If your patient doesn't have an I.V. line in place, establish one at keep-vein-open (KVO) rate.

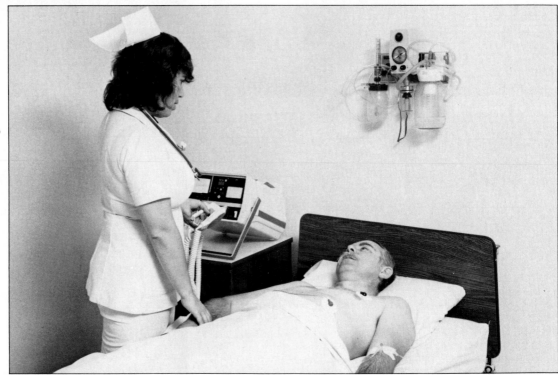

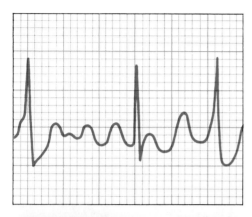

3 Run an EKG rhythm strip to determine that he still has atrial flutter.

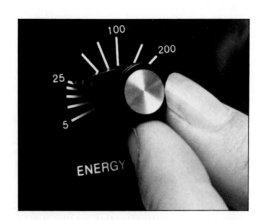

7 Set the control panel to the correct number of joules or watt-seconds, as indicated by the doctor.

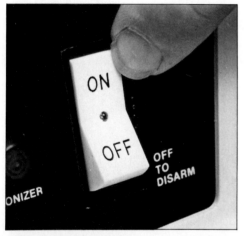

4 Plug in the defibrillator and turn it on.
 Most doctors will want to administer a premedication, such as Valium I.V. If your patient's doctor has done so, prepare the medication for administration. Have a hand-held resuscitator ready to give your patient respiratory support.

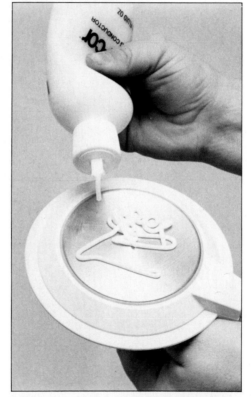

8 Apply a generous amount of conductive jelly to each paddle. Coat the surface of each paddle with jelly by rubbing them together. Remove any excess jelly after you separate the paddles.

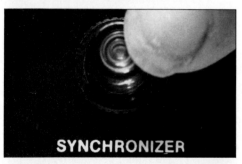

5 Set the defibrillator on the cardiovert mode by depressing the SYNCHRONIZER button. From now on, we'll refer to the defibrillator as a cardioverter.

6 Examine the EKG rhythm strip again. The R wave should be at least 3 cm high. If it isn't, turn the ECG SIZE (gain) knob until it is. The R wave must be this tall to trigger the cardioverter. Only with this triggering can the cardioverter deliver a synchronized shock at the proper time.

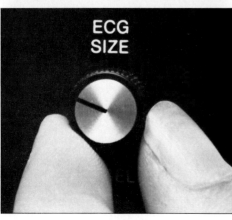

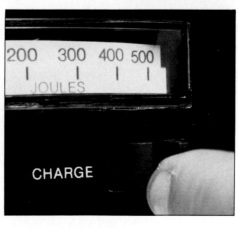

9 Then, push the charge button on the cardioverter until the display number matches the joules or watt-second setting.

Emergency procedures

Performing cardioversion continued

10 The doctor will position the paddles as he would for defibrillation: one paddle on the right side of the sternum below the clavicle, and the other on the left side of the chest, at the midclavicular line, fifth intercostal space. If your patient's a child or the paddles are different from those shown here, the doctor will place one paddle on the anterior chest, left of the sternum, and the other on the posterior chest below the shoulder blades.

11 When the doctor's ready to cardiovert, he'll warn everyone to step back from the patient and the bed. This way, no one will be accidentally shocked. Then, he'll simultaneously press the buttons on both paddles. The cardioverter will automatically deliver the shock on the next R wave of the patient's EKG. After the shock is administered, the doctor will remove the paddles from the patient's chest.

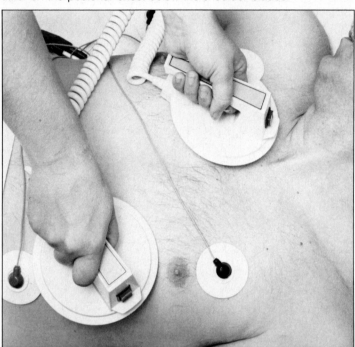

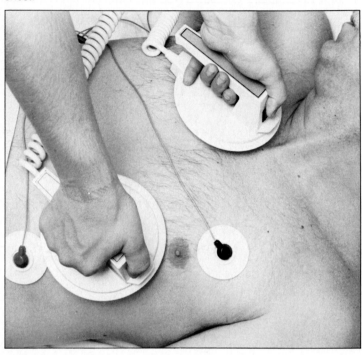

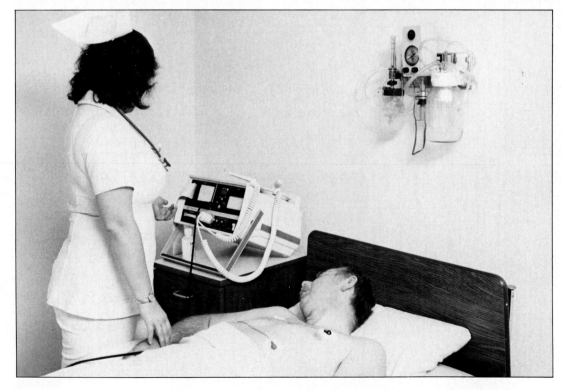

12 Check the patient's vital signs and gauge his responsiveness. Then, examine the EKG strip to determine if the cardioversion was successful. If it wasn't, the doctor may want to repeat the procedure.

If repeating the procedure is unnecessary, turn off the cardioverter's power. Clean the paddles with soap and water to keep them from corroding. Document the entire procedure, as well as your observations, in your nurses' notes.

Using an automatic rotating tourniquet machine

1 *Fifty-eight-year-old Allen Marley has pulmonary edema, according to his doctor's diagnosis. As you know, that means fluid has accumulated in his lung tissue. To combat the condition, the doctor administered potent diuretics. While he's waiting for the drugs to take effect, he decides to try reducing blood flow to Mr. Marley's heart by impeding venous return from his arms and legs. That's why he instructs you to apply rotating tourniquets. Do you know how? The procedure's not difficult, especially if your hospital has an automatic rotating tourniquet machine. (If it doesn't have this machine,* turn to page 99 to learn how to *rotate tourniquets manually.)*

You'll need this equipment: an automatic rotating tourniquet machine and four small towels (not shown).

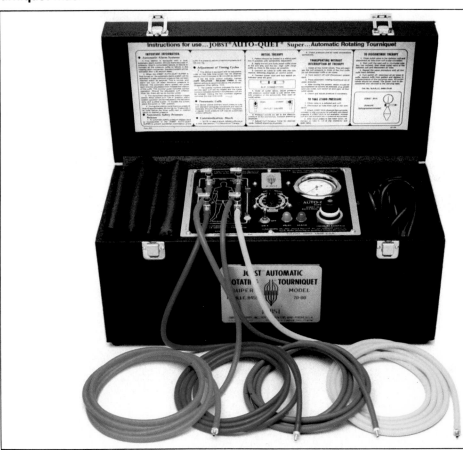

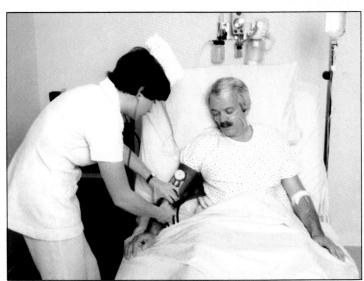

2 Begin by explaining the procedure to your patient. Tell him that the tourniquets may be uncomfortable and that his arms and legs might temporarily swell or discolor. Answer all his questions before proceeding.

Then, place the patient in Fowler's position. Record his blood pressure, heart and respiratory rates, and radial and pedal pulse rates.

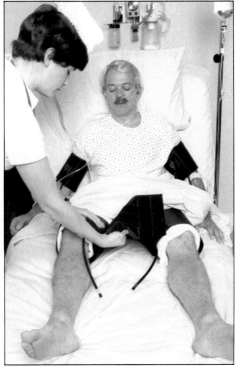

3 Wrap a towel and tourniquet around each of his arms and legs, about 4" (10 cm) from his axillae and 4" (10 cm) from his groin. Apply the tourniquets snugly enough to allow only two fingers to be inserted between the tourniquet and skin.

Note: Obviously, the nurse in this photo will make sure that the patient's peripheral I.V. line is replaced with a central I.V. line. If she didn't, blood would back into the peripheral I.V. line and clog it.

Emergency procedures

Using an automatic rotating tourniquet machine continued

4 Then, connect the tourniquet hoses to their color-coded mates on the machine.

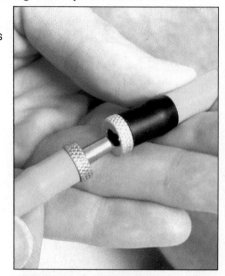

5 Make sure the machine's turned off. Then, close the tourniquet inflation valves, as the nurse is doing here. When the valves are closed, turn on the machine.

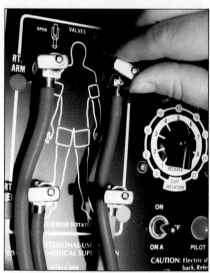

6 Set the machine's pressure dial, as ordered by the doctor. You'll probably set it somewhere between 40 and 60 mm Hg, depending on your patient's blood pressure.

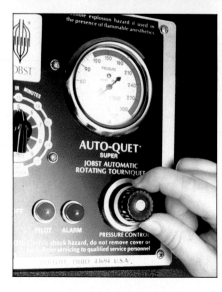

7 Set the inflation timing mechanism, as ordered (usually about 15 minutes).

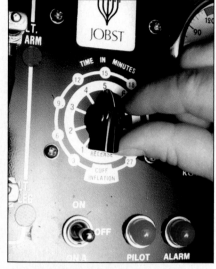

8 Open the tourniquet valves. Three of the four tourniquets will automatically inflate. Then, every 15 minutes (in a clockwise cycle), one of those tourniquets will deflate, and the previously deflated tourniquet will inflate. At no time are all four tourniquets inflated. As the therapy progresses, make sure the tourniquets are inflating in proper clockwise order.

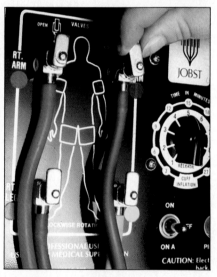

9 Regularly assess the patient's arms and legs below the inflated tourniquets for color, temperature, and pulse. Also, check the patient's heart and lung sounds and measure his blood pressure frequently. Notify the doctor of any abnormalities.

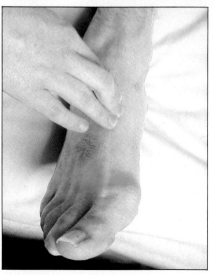

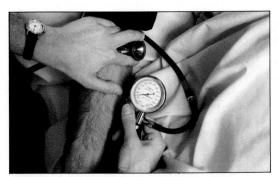

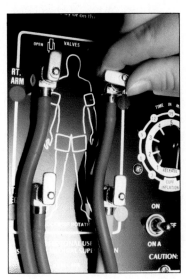

10 Here's an easy way to take the blood pressure of a patient on a rotating tourniquet machine. Disconnect the *uninflated* tourniquet from the machine tubing. Connect the special blood pressure sphygmomanometer (supplied by the manufacturer) to the tourniquet and proceed as usual.

11 When the doctor has determined that the patient's pulmonary edema has been effectively treated, close the inflation valve of the uninflated tourniquet. Remove that tourniquet from the patient's arm or leg. Assess that extremity for changes in the rate and character of the arterial pulse, and the temperature and color of the skin. Note your findings. Monitor the patient's vital signs closely during weaning, to make sure he doesn't need the tourniquets anymore.

As each of the other tourniquets deflate at 15 minute intervals, close their corresponding inflation valves and remove them. Gradually discontinuing the process in this way prevents a sudden increase in the patient's venous blood volume, which could cause circulatory overload.

Finally, document the procedure, the time you started and ended, and your observations, particularly those regarding swelling or discoloration.

Rotating tourniquets manually

Perhaps your hospital doesn't own an automatic rotating tourniquet machine, or suppose the machine's in use when you need it. What do you do? You'll have to rotate the tourniquets manually. In this piece, we'll review the basics of this procedure. But, if you want detailed instruction, see the NURSING PHOTOBOOK *Dealing with Emergencies.*

First, gather three towels and three blood pressure cuffs, which we'll refer to as tourniquets. Follow the same tourniquet application procedure we described in the preceding story, but leave one extremity free.

Inflate each tourniquet to the pressure ordered by the doctor, checking for snugness using the two-finger method described on page 97. Wait 15 minutes. Then, moving clockwise, deflate and remove the tourniquet and towel nearest the free extremity.

Place the towel and tourniquet on the formerly free extremity. Inflate the tourniquet and check for snugness. Repeat this rotation procedure every 15 minutes, using the timing and suggested pattern outlined in this illustration. Post the rotation plan at your patient's bedside and follow it carefully.

Remove the tourniquets as you would with an automatic rotating tourniquet machine. The only difference is you don't have to turn off any inflation valve.

Finally, document the procedure in your nurses' notes.

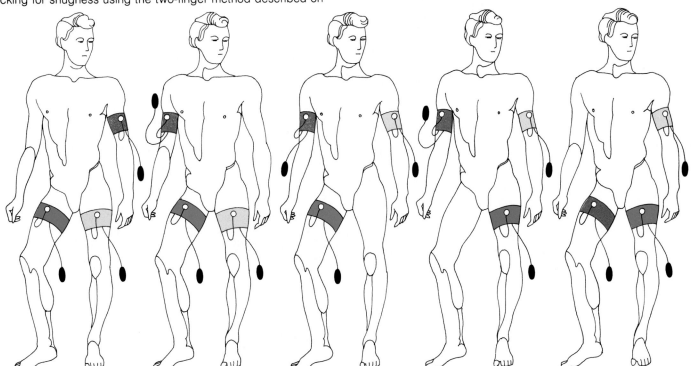

Emergency procedures

Learning about the intra-aortic balloon pump (IABP)

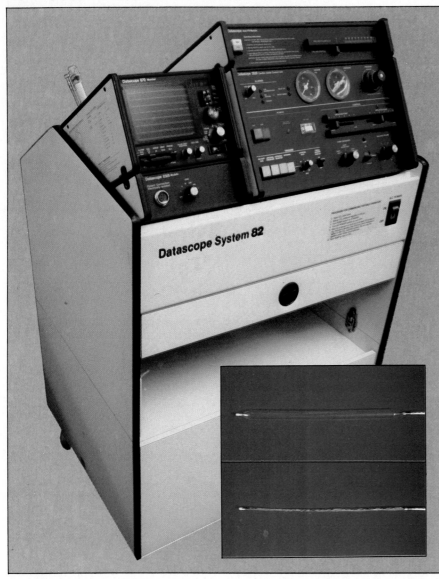

Datascope System 82

You probably know what an intra-aortic balloon pump (IABP) is, but do you know why a balloon is inserted and how it improves cardiac efficiency? The IABP assists a weakened or damaged left ventricle, helping to increase coronary artery perfusion and aiding left ventricular ejection. Here's how it works:

An intra-aortic balloon (see inset) is just that—a balloon about 10″ (25 cm) long, made of antithrombogenic material, and consisting of one, two, or three chambers. It's mounted on the distal end of a semiflexible catheter that's connected to a pump console.

The balloon's inserted through the patient's femoral artery, either surgically (using a cutdown procedure and a vein graft), or percutaneously. Surgical insertion is still common, but percutaneous insertion will become more and more prevalent because the procedure:
• requires a minimal amount of equipment.
• can be performed rapidly.
• can be performed by any doctor, not just a cardio-vascular surgeon.
• avoids the risks of sepsis and erosion.

Also, when weaning's completed, a balloon inserted percutaneously is much easier to remove than one inserted surgically.

After insertion, the balloon's tip is positioned in the aorta, just below the left subclavian artery. Placement is confirmed by fluoroscopy or X-ray.

The pump console monitors the patient's heartbeat. The R wave in the EKG pattern triggers the pump's inflating mechanism, which then sends carbon dioxide or helium into the balloon. Carbon dioxide is commonly used, but some manufacturers recommend helium because it's lighter, which makes for quicker balloon inflation/deflation.

As the balloon inflates, it displaces blood. This displacement increases aortic blood pressure, which enhances coronary blood flow. Then, as the heart prepares for left ventricular ejection, the balloon deflates, decreasing aortic blood pressure. This makes ejection easier, decreasing the left ventricle's workload.

Using the intra-aortic balloon pump (IABP)

The doctor may insert an intra-aortic balloon (IAB) when your patient has:
• cardiogenic shock
• unsuccessful weaning from cardiopulmonary bypass machine
• myocardial infarction
• ventricular septal defect
• acute mitral valve regurgitation
• myocardial ischemia
• preinfarction angina.
    He won't insert an IAB if your patient has:
• aortic aneurysm
• moderate to severe aortic valvular insufficiency
• peripheral vascular disease.
• terminal disease.

Learning about an external counterpulsation technique

What's external pressure circulatory assist? It's a noninvasive counterpulsation technique that's used to treat cardiac failure.

This is how it works: Water-filled pumping chambers, placed on each of your patient's legs, pump up and down in synchronization with your patient's cardiac cycle. During diastole, the chambers apply 250 mm Hg of positive pressure to the legs. During systole, the chambers empty and apply 50 mm Hg of negative pressure. This pumping action alters peripheral blood volume and modifies aortic pressure. Studies also show external counterpulsation enhances coronary circulation.

How does external pressure circulatory assist compare with the intra-aortic balloon pump (IABP)? The counterpulsation technique doesn't reduce afterload as effectively as the IABP. But, like IABP, external counterpulsation can't be used if the patient has aortic valve insufficiency or peripheral artery or venous disease. Also, as happens with an IABP, this procedure may cause your patient discomfort.

Helping with a surgical intra-aortic balloon insertion

An intra-aortic balloon can be inserted surgically or percutaneously. Since percutaneous insertion is quickly becoming the method of choice among most doctors, we've chosen to spotlight that technique in the following photostory. But before we do, we thought we'd review the basics of surgical insertion and your role in the procedure.

• A doctor may perform surgical insertion in the OR or at the patient's bedside. If he chooses the patient's bedside, you'll need to set up a mini OR there. Many hospitals have a balloon pump cart that can be wheeled wherever it's needed. It would include most of this equipment: umbilical tape, vascular scissors, a piece of ⅜″ (1 cm) woven Dacron® or Teflon® graft, an emesis basin, 5,000 units heparin I.V., 500 ml sterile saline solution, 50 cc syringe, 50 cc Xylocaine 1% without epinephrine, stopcock, intra-aortic balloon catheter, and IABP console. In addition, obtain the following: a defibrillator, intubation equipment, emergency medication, infusion pump, two oxygen outlets, two vacuum outlets, and a unit of typed and cross-matched blood. Make sure these items are in place: a cardiac monitor, a peripheral I.V. line, a pulmonary artery line, a peripheral arterial line, and possibly another central arterial line.

• All personnel must be masked, capped, gloved, and gowned. You must maintain strict aseptic technique throughout the procedure, especially when you touch surgical packs and instruments.

• Before the doctor can insert the intra-aortic balloon, he must explain the procedure to the patient or his family and ask for formal consent. Make sure the patient understands the procedure so he's prepared for every step. Keep in mind that he won't be able to move and may experience pain during the procedure. So, provide the reassurance and emotional support he needs.

• Then, plug in the IABP console. You'll find the console is also equipped with a cable that can be plugged into the cardiac monitor. When connected, an EKG waveform appears simultaneously on the cardiac monitor and the IABP console. Because the EKG waveform will not be used for diagnostic purposes but rather as a device for triggering balloon action, make sure you choose the lead in which the R wave is dominant. It must be at least 3 cm (1¼″) . tall to trigger balloon inflation.

• Check and record the patient's peripheral pulses. Tell the doctor about any abnormalities, especially in popliteal or dorsalis pedis pulses. If your patient's not fully conscious, also do a baseline neurologic check.

• Uncover the patient's groin and prep both sides with an alcohol swab and povidone-iodine solution. Then, as the doctor prepares for the arteriotomy, program the IABP console, following the manufacturer's instructions and the doctor's orders.

• Then, open the balloon package carefully, maintaining sterility, and drop it on a sterile field. The doctor will test the balloon for defects and ready it for insertion.

• About 3 minutes before the doctor performs the arteriotomy, he will usually order the administration of an anticoagulant, such as heparin 5,000 u. Follow his instructions.

• Meanwhile, the doctor will prepare the site for incision, expose the femoral artery, and then clamp it, so he can perform the arteriotomy.

At this point, the patient may feel some discomfort, such as leg numbness. If, at any time during the procedure, the patient complains of pain, notify the doctor. He may order a drug, such as morphine sulfate, to treat it. If the patient suffers an acute sudden back pain during insertion (a sign of dissection), the doctor will discontinue the procedure.

• After the doctor performs the arteriotomy, he'll place a graft over the balloon and catheter. Then, he'll thread the balloon up the

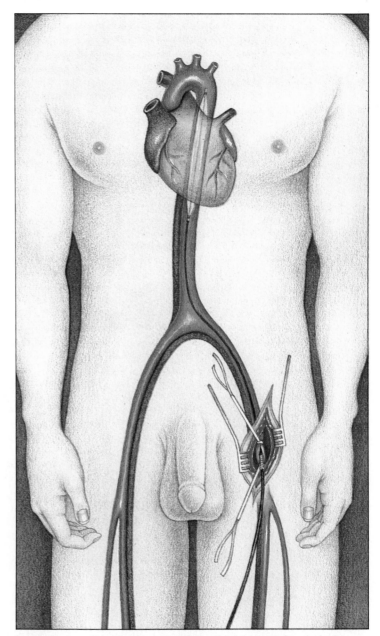

femoral artery, into the thoracic aorta distal to the left subclavian artery. When that's completed, he'll suture a side arm graft to the arteriotomy and to the exposed catheter. This will help provide circulation to the leg below the balloon catheter. With a portable chest X-ray or fluoroscope, he'll check the balloon's position. If all's well, the doctor will suture the balloon catheter into place and close the incision.

• Now, attach the balloon catheter to the IABP console. The console operator will turn on the pump and check inflation/deflation timing.

• Cover the insertion site with antibacterial ointment. Then, with sterile scissors, make a small cut into one side of an occlusive bandage. Place the bandage over the insertion site so that the catheter extends out of the small cut.

• Finally, document the procedure in your nurses' notes.

Emergency procedures

Assisting with percutaneous intra-aortic balloon insertion

1 *Have you ever assisted with an intra-aortic balloon insertion? If you have, the doctor probably inserted the balloon surgically. But now there's a new, better way: percutaneous insertion. To learn all about it, read on.*

First, you'll be responsible for gathering this equipment: an 18G angiographic needle; a .038x125 cm safety J guide; a Datascope PERCOR™ percutaneous introducer dilator and sheath; a 50 cc syringe; a basin filled with sterile saline solution; a No. 8 French dilator; umbilical tape; a 3-way stopcock; and lidocaine. Place all equipment on a tray to carry it to the bedside. Make sure you maintain sterile technique in handling all equipment.

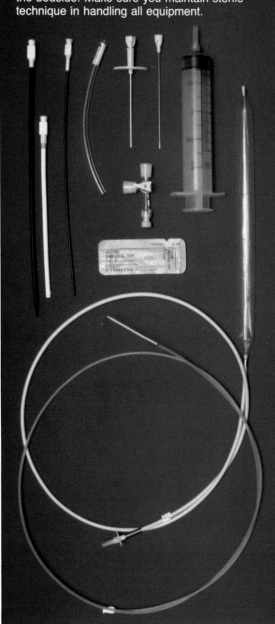

2 Uncover the patient's groin and prep the right side with an alcohol swab and povidone-iodine solution. Then, the doctor will use the angiographic needle to puncture the anterior wall of the femoral artery. After he inserts the safety J guide into the needle, he'll remove the needle and make a small incision where the safety guide exits the skin. Next, he'll insert the No. 8 French dilator through the skin, over the safety J guide, to dilate the vessel. Then, he'll remove the No. 8 French dilator and exchange it for the PERCOR™ percutaneous introducer dilator and sheath, leaving the safety J guide in place.

Important: The doctor may ask you to hold the introducer and safety J guide in place for the remainder of the procedure. If they're not held in place, high blood pressure may expel them from the artery.

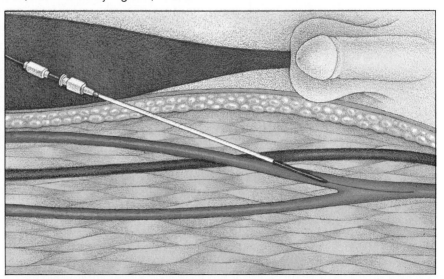

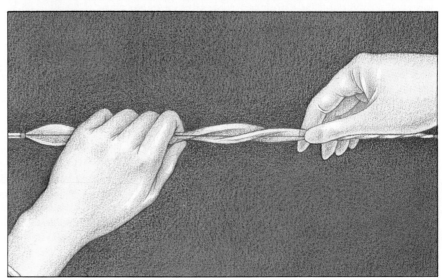

3 Now the doctor will ask you to unwrap the intra-aortic balloon. He'll take the balloon and place the wrapping indicator on its tip. This serves as his guide when he wraps the balloon. Next, he'll insert the wrapping indicator and balloon into the sterile saline solution. (He may add lidocaine to the solution to minimize local arterial spasm upon insertion and to aid lubrication.) Then, he'll grasp the wrapping indicator in one hand and the balloon in the other. He'll begin turning the wrapping indicator clockwise, until he's turned it nine times.

4 He'll hold the balloon so it remains twisted as you attach a 3-way stopcock to the end of the balloon catheter. Then, attach a 50 cc syringe to the 3-way stopcock.

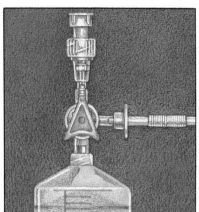

5 Turn the stopcock off to the open port and draw back on the syringe plunger. This draws out all air from the balloon and creates a vacuum. Turn the stopcock so it's off to the balloon catheter. This maintains the vacuum and allows you to remove the syringe.

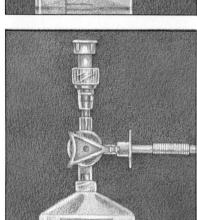

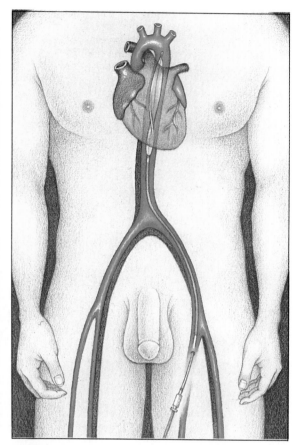

7 Then, he'll remove the safety J guide and the introducer dilator, leaving just the PERCOR™ transcutaneous introducer sheath at the insertion site. He'll begin feeding the intra-aortic balloon into the introducer sheath, rotating the balloon clockwise to make sure that the balloon remains tightly wrapped. He'll position the balloon just below the left subclavian artery and confirm placement by radiography.

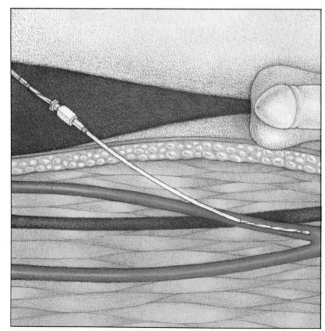

6 Just before insertion, begin administering the ordered anticoagulant intravenously. The doctor will remove the wrapping indicator and immerse the balloon in sterile saline solution once more.

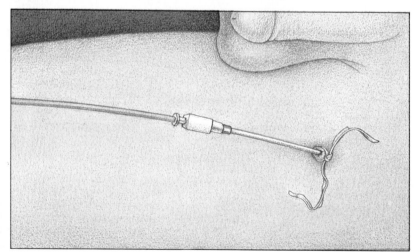

8 Remove the stopcock from the catheter tip to release the vacuum. The balloon will unwrap by itself. Place an umbilical tape snare around the introducer to control bleeding from the site. The doctor will connect the catheter to the preprogrammed IABP console, and press the appropriate button to prefill the balloon. Pumping can now commence.

Palpate the femoral artery distal to the insertion site. If the pulse is weak or absent, tell the doctor. He may establish a time limit for the therapy. If the femoral artery is too deep to palpate, then palpate the posterior popliteal or dorsalis pedis instead. Document the procedure in your nurses' notes.

Emergency procedures

Caring for the patient on an intra-aortic balloon pump (IABP)

What are your responsibilities in managing the patient on an intra-aortic balloon pump? Follow the doctor's specific instructions for each patient's care, but study the following list to understand the basics:
• Take your patient's baseline vital signs and neurologic signs before the procedure, then every 15 minutes afterward until the patient is stable. At that time, you can take them once each hour.
• In addition, assess the following at least once an hour: your patient's cardiac rhythm (which is being monitored continuously), cardiac output, urinary output, pulmonary artery pressure (PAP), and the arterial pulse, temperature, and skin color of the leg with the insertion site.
• Assess pulmonary artery wedge pressure (PAWP) every four hours.
• Change the dressing on the insertion site once a day, or as ordered (following your hospital's procedure.) Check the site for signs of bleeding, inflammation, or infection.
• Inspect the balloon catheter regularly for signs of kinking or cracking. Make sure the catheter pump joint is connected securely.
• Check the EKG occasionally to make sure the R wave remains large enough to trigger the balloon pump. Eliminate any artifacts. Also, examine the arterial pressure wave and adjust inflation or deflation timing, if necessary.
• Draw arterial blood samples, as the doctor orders.
• Don't allow your patient to bend at the

Reading arterial pressure waves

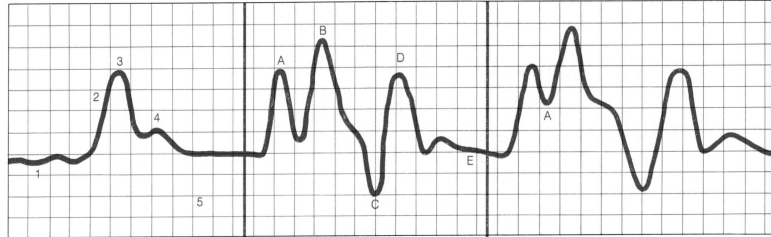

An important part of caring for the patient on an intra-aortic balloon pump (IABP) is maintaining the proper timing of inflation and deflation.

You can't use an EKG to determine whether or not the timing is accurate, because the EKG is an *electric signal*. The balloon's action must be correlated with aortic pressure, represented by the *hemodynamic signal*. That's why the IABP console also features an aortic pressure signal.

Pictured above is a normal arterial pressure tracing:
1. Aortic valve opens, ventricular ejection occurs.
2. Maximal ejection period.
3. Peak of systolic phase.
4. Aortic valve closure (dicrotic notch); diastole begins.
5. Diastole ends.

When a balloon is introduced into the aorta, its inflation and deflation significantly affect the tracing. The following tracings will show you how.

The above tracing shows good balloon timing. Pictured are two complete systolic and diastolic events. This tracing demonstrates that after the peak of systole (A), the balloon inflates at the point where the dicrotic notch is usually seen, causing a rise in diastolic pressure to B, its peak. The balloon then deflates at the end of diastole and reduces the aortic diastolic pressure (C). This reduction in end diastolic pressure can be clearly seen by comparing C to E. E shows that normal end diastolic pressure is higher when there is no balloon deflation. Also note the slight reduction in systolic pressure following deflation (D). As the illustration above shows, timing is good when:
• inflation takes place at the dicrotic notch.
• assisted diastolic pressure is higher than the systolic pressure (in certain special circumstances it will not be higher).
• assisted end diastolic pressure is less than the end diastolic pressure without balloon assistance (usually about 10 to 15 mm Hg reduction in end diastole).
• systolic pressure is slightly reduced following balloon deflation.

The above tracing shows *early inflation*. Early inflation (A) increases intra-aortic pressure. This causes early closure of the aortic valve, before ejection is complete, and leaves the left ventricle partially filled.

waist more than 45°. Never *flex* the affected leg, at the hip or the knee, although other movement of that leg, such as ankle exercises with a foot board, is beneficial. Treat him as if he were in a long body spica cast. Turn him by logrolling. Allow him to stand to urinate, if his doctor says it's okay.
• As your patient improves, the doctor may order weaning. This will involve reducing the IAB pumping ratio until the patient's heart can function without assistance. Because of the nature of IABP therapy, expect the weaning process to be very gradual. Be particularly alert for signs of deterioration in your patient. If you detect any, notify the doctor and he'll alter the weaning procedure.

Important: If the balloon pump fails, take steps to keep the balloon in motion while the pump is being fixed or another is being located. For example, some pumps have a flutter feature, which, when used, keeps the balloon moving slightly. If this feature isn't operating, or isn't available, detach the connector tubing from the pump and connect a syringe to the tubing. Every 5 minutes, rapidly inflate and deflate the balloon with small amounts of air. By keeping the balloon in motion, you prevent blood from clotting in the folds of the balloon membrane.

Caution: Don't do this flutter procedure if the console indicates the balloon's broken or leaking, or if you see blood in the balloon catheter. Instead, call the doctor immediately.

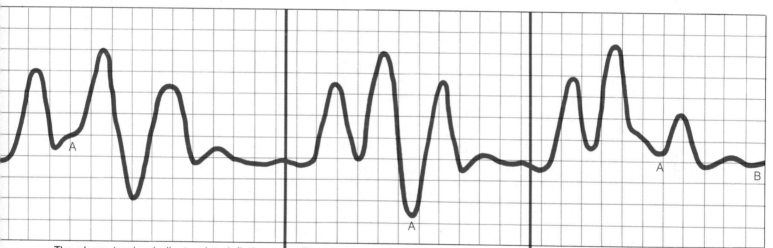

The above tracing indicates *late inflation.* The dicrotic notch (A) is clearly visible, which means aortic pressure remains low for too long, causing inefficient arterial perfusion. The inflation control on the console should be adjusted so that inflation takes place earlier, at the dicrotic notch.

The above tracing shows *early deflation.* By having the balloon deflate prior to contraction, the benefit of decreased afterload is lost. Adjust the deflation control to compensate. There also may be retrograde flow from the coronary arteries. Note the configuration of the end diastolic curve of balloon deflation (A) and compare it to a good tracing. Also note there's no visible reduction in the systole following balloon deflation.

This tracing reflects *late deflation,* because the end diastolic pressure (A) created by balloon deflation is higher than the end diastolic pressure without balloon assistance (B). This tells you that the balloon is staying inflated too long, keeping aortic pressure high. This increases myocardial work. The deflation control on the console should be adjusted so that deflation takes place earlier.

Important: Remember that not all waveforms look alike. Examine each waveform for individual landmarks.

Emergency procedures

Troubleshooting intra-aortic balloon pump (IABP) therapy

Problem	Possible cause	Solution
Balloon is inflating too frequently or erratically	• Patient has a pacemaker	• Manipulate EKG leads so you get a dominant R wave and minimized pacemaker spike. • Set the pacemaker on the lowest threshold level. • Switch to arterial pressure triggering.
	• Patient has multiple atrial arrhythmias	• Treat arrhythmias, per doctor's orders. • Set timing to the most common R-R interval (preferably short) while treating arrhythmias.
	• Artifact on EKG tracing caused by the equipment	• Eliminate artifact or switch to arterial pressure triggering.
Augmentation curve (pressure curve caused by balloon inflation) is absent or too small	• Pump turned off	• Turn on the pump.
	• No gas in balloon	• Check gas supply and refill, if necessary. • Check tubing for kinks and connections for leaks. Notify doctor, if you detect any. • Following the manufacturer's instructions, check balloon for leaks. If you find any, the doctor will replace the balloon.
	• Arterial pressure may be damped	• Check arterial pressure tubing and connections for air bubbles, kinks, or leaks. Flush, if necessary.
	• Patient is hypovolemic	• Notify doctor. Treat hypovolemia, as ordered.
	• Patient's cardiac stroke volume exceeds balloon volume	• Notify doctor. He'll probably begin weaning the patient from the balloon pump.
	• Balloon positioned too low in aorta or in a false channel of the aorta	• Notify doctor. He may remove or reposition the balloon.
Augmentation curve is too large	• Too much gas entering balloon	• Decrease gas flow.
	• Balloon too large for patient	• Notify doctor. He may replace balloon with a smaller one.
Balloon is deflating prematurely	• Patient has frequent premature ventricular contractions (PVCs)	• Treat arrhythmias.
Balloon loses gas pressure more quickly than the anticipated gradual loss	• Balloon leak	• Stop pumping to investigate. • Check connections. Following manufacturer's guidelines, check balloon for leaks. Notify the doctor, if you find any.
Balloon inflation alarm sounds	• Depleted gas supply	• Reload the gas system, if necessary. • Increase the balloon inflation pressure so that it reaches at least +50 mm Hg.
High volume alarm sounds	• Balloon pump volume meter setting exceeds the capacity of balloon	• Check the volume meter setting. Decrease the setting, if necessary, so it matches the balloon volume.
	• Balloon catheter improperly connected to console	• Reconnect the balloon catheter to the console.
Arterial pressure is absent or too low	• Disconnected balloon catheter or pressure transducer	• Check and secure all connections.
Arterial pressure is too high, exceeding 200 mm Hg	• Improperly calibrated pressure transducer	• Recalibrate the transducer, following the procedure outlined in the NURSING PHOTOBOOK Using Monitors.
Arterial pressure waveform is damped	• Blocked arterial pressure catheter	• Flush the arterial pressure catheter.
Arterial pressure waveform is obscured by interference	• Patient movement	• Quiet the patient.
	• Jostled catheter	• Eliminate any disturbances.

Cardiac pacemakers

The patient who needs help maintaining his cardiac rhythm needs help fast. That's what a pacemaker's for. If the doctor orders a pacemaker for your patient, he may ask you to assist him with the insertion. Learn all you can about the procedure.

Your most important roles, however, are preparing the patient for the insertion and giving him special care and competent instruction after the insertion. Find out how to provide these things for your patient by reading the following pages.

When your patient needs a cardiac pacemaker

An electrocardiogram (EKG) of your patient's heart is a doctor's best tool in determining whether or not your patient needs a cardiac pacemaker. If he decides the patient needs a pacemaker, the doctor can order either a temporary or permanent one, depending on the situation. For example, a temporary pacemaker is inserted if the patient's cardiac abnormality is an emergency, such as asystole, or is transient, such as drug toxicopathy or an inferior wall myocardial infarction. A permanent pacemaker's inserted if the patient's cardiac problem is a rhythm abnormality, such as one of those listed here:
• sinus bradycardia (when the SA node fires less than 60 times per minute)
• sinus arrest (when the SA node fails to fire consistently)
• atrial fibrillation with a slow ventricular response (when the SA node fires rapidly but the AV junction blocks some of the impulses)
• second-degree AV block (when the SA node impulses do not consistently reach the ventricles)
• complete heart block (when the AV junction blocks all SA node impulses)
• bifascicular bundle branch block (when the electrical impulses are blocked at the right bundle branch or segments of the left bundle branch)
• ventricular tachycardia (when the ventricle repeatedly contracts prematurely)
• sinus pause (when the SA node fails to fire rhythmically)
• bradytachycardia (when the SA node fires more rapidly and then more slowly than normal)

Learning about cardiac pacemakers

All cardiac pacing systems have two main components: the pacer (or pulse generator), and the electrode. First, in this chart, let's examine the two types of pacemakers available, temporary and permanent, and the batteries that power them. On the following pages, we'll take a closer look at the pacers themselves and the electrodes used with them.

Type of pacemaker	Purpose	Placement	Power source	Life expectancy	Special information
Temporary	For short-term cardiac pacing	External pacer; internal electrode	Rechargeable or replaceable batteries	2 weeks of continuous use	• Check and replace periodically, even when not in use. • Keep replacement directions handy • Do not immerse pacer in any liquid
Permanent	For long-term cardiac pacing	Internal pacer and electrode	Mercury-zinc	3 to 4 years	• Rarely used today
			Lithium	3 to 15 years	• Several variations of the lithium battery available (most common: lithium-iodide)
			Nuclear	20 to 40 years	• Power source life expectancy depends on half-life of radioactive material in the battery • Battery under Nuclear Regulatory Commission supervision

Cardiac pacemakers

Understanding pacers

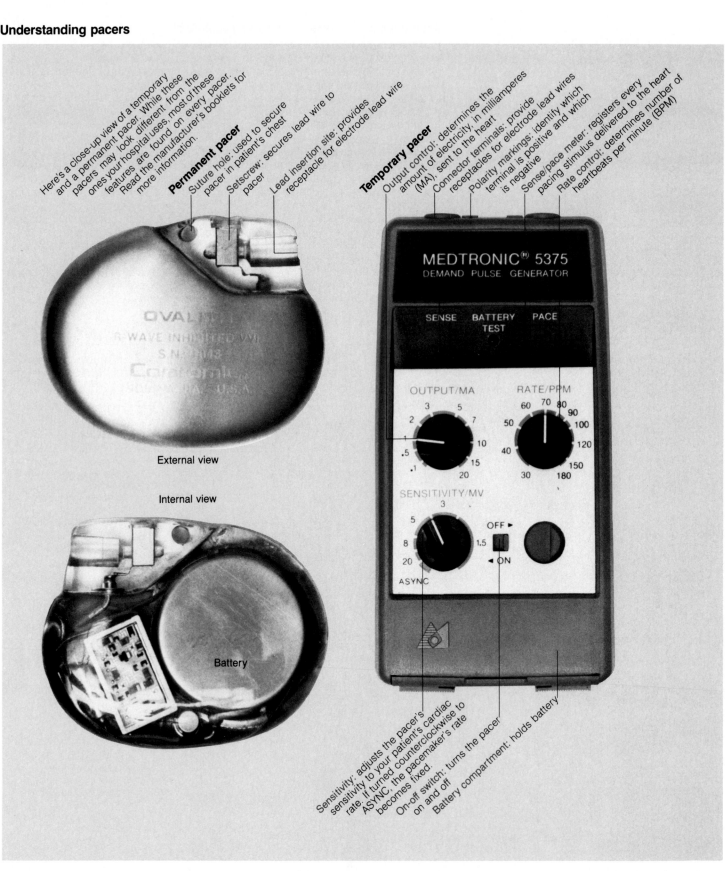

Here's a close-up view of a temporary and a permanent pacer. While these pacers may look different from the ones your hospital uses, most of these features are found on every pacer. Read the manufacturer's booklets for more information.

Permanent pacer

Suture hole: used to secure pacer in patient's chest

Setscrew: secures lead wire to pacer

Lead insertion site: provides receptacle for electrode lead wire

Temporary pacer

Output control: determines the amount of electricity, in milliamperes (MA), sent to the heart

Connector terminals: provide receptacles for electrode lead wires

Polarity markings: identify which terminal is positive and which is negative

Sense/pace meter: registers every pacing stimulus delivered to the heart

Rate control: determines number of heartbeats per minute (BPM)

External view

Internal view

Battery

Sensitivity: adjusts the pacer's sensitivity to your patient's cardiac rate. If turned counterclockwise to ASYNC, the pacemaker's rate becomes fixed.

On-off switch: turns the pacer on and off

Battery compartment: holds battery

MEDTRONIC 5375
DEMAND PULSE GENERATOR

SENSE   BATTERY   PACE
TEST

OUTPUT/MA   RATE/PPM

SENSITIVITY/MV

OFF ▶

◀ ON

ASYNC

Learning about pacing electrodes

The pacing electrode is the part of the pacemaker system that runs from the pacer into the heart. It transmits the patient's cardiac rhythm to the pacer. The pacer then delivers a stimulus to the heart via this same electrode. Two main types of electrodes are now in use: unipolar and bipolar.

Electrical current can flow only when there's a positive and negative pole. The *unipolar* electrode gets its name from the single pole imbedded in its tip. The other pole that's necessary for electrical conduction is built into the casing of the implanted pacer. The unipolar electrode pro-

duces tall EKG pacing spikes because of the distance between the two poles.

The *bipolar* electrode has both poles imbedded in the electrode itself: one pole in the tip and the other pole, an exposed metal ring, about an inch farther up the electrode lead wire. The bipolar electrode produces short EKG pacing spikes because the two poles are so close together.

Many styles of electrode tips are available. Which one the doctor selects depends on the mode of pacing and the insertion site. Below are some examples of typical electrode tips.

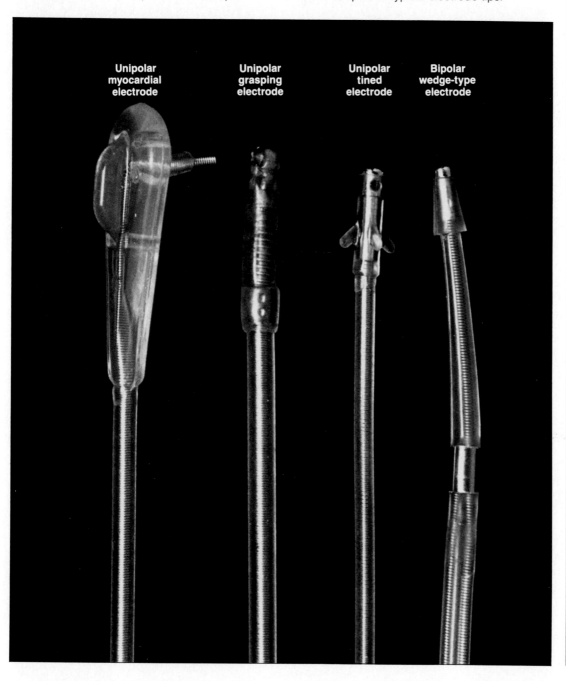

Unipolar myocardial electrode   **Unipolar grasping electrode**   **Unipolar tined electrode**   **Bipolar wedge-type electrode**

Learning pacemaker terminology

When you're caring for a patient with a pacemaker, you should know common pacemaker terminology. Read the following cases to familiarize yourself with several of those terms.

• The doctor asks you to help him establish your patient's cardiac *threshold*. Do you know what he means? Threshold refers to the minimum amount of electrical current produced by the pacemaker necessary to stimulate cardiac repolarization. On the EKG, you'll see the pacemaker spike, followed by a QRS complex.

• In examining your patient's EKG, you clearly see the pacemaker spike but no QRS complex. A coworker says she suspects the problem is *loss of capture*. What does she mean? Loss of capture occurs when the pacemaker fires, but the heart's not stimulated.

• The doctor tells you the demand pacemaker's *sensing capability* is malfunctioning. What does that mean? Sensing capability refers to the pacemaker's ability to sense electrical stimulation in the heart. When the SA node fails to fire on its own, the sensing mechanism tells the pacemaker to fire in its stead. The sensing capability is malfunctioning when the SA node fails to fire and the pacemaker doesn't fire either.

• The doctor chooses a demand pacemaker over a fixed one, explaining he wants to avoid *competition*. What is he talking about? Competition, in the case of a fixed pacemaker, means the firing of the pacemaker competes with the patient's intrinsic beat. Competition may also occur with a demand pacemaker, when the pacemaker's sensing mechanism is malfunctioning and the pacemaker fires at random.

Cardiac pacemakers

Preparing the patient for pacemaker insertion

If your patient is like most, needing a pacemaker scares him. But, a pacemaker isn't dangerous. In fact, it can give your patient many more active years of life. Help him accept the idea by adequately preparing him for pacemaker insertion (which we'll discuss here), and for living with his pacemaker (which we'll discuss later).

First, your patient's surgeon and cardiologist will discuss the pacemaker with him. Those discussions may raise questions in your patient's mind about how his heart works. Then, if he wants to learn more, provide him with helpful, illustrated booklets published by the American Heart Association and pacemaker manufacturers. If possible, examine the booklets with him.

Perhaps he'd like to see a pacer. Show him a demonstration unit and review how the pacemaker works. By talking with your patient, you may find out that he's afraid the pacemaker may stop unexpectedly. Clear up his misconceptions.

Next, describe the insertion procedure, telling him what will be done and showing him where the pacer will be inserted. Answer all of his questions honestly.

To learn more about how you can help the patient with a pacemaker, read the patient teaching information on page 117.

Nurses' guide to pacemaker mode and placement

Years ago, differentiating pacemaker modes was easy. The pacemaker was set to fire into a patient's ventricle either at a fixed rate or at a demand rate. But today, pacemaker modes and placement are not so simple. Of course, you may still employ fixed or demand pacemakers. But you'll probably use a variation or combination of these basic modes, such as a pacemaker that senses one chamber, but fires at a fixed rate into another (Demand example B). Or you may use a new mode entirely, such as a physiological pacemaker that fires into the atrium and ventricle, as needed, to synchronize right-sided heart contractions.

Several ways exist to differentiate pacemakers. Each manufacturer assigns its own designations to its pacemakers. Your hospital may use those designations. Or your hospital may identify pacemaker types and operating modes by using a letter code. Codes vary from hospital to hospital, so if your hospital employs one, make sure you learn it.

This chart features basic pacemaker modes and a few variations. To learn about your patient's pacemaker, consult the manufacturer's booklet.

Pacemaker mode	Description	Electrode placement
FIXED (example A)	Pacemaker delivers an electrical impulse at a predetermined rate to the atrium or the ventricle (depending on electrode placement). Pacemaker rate remains fixed regardless of the patient's intrinsic heart rate.	Right ventricle or, in rare cases, right atrium (not shown)
DEMAND (example A)	Pacemaker senses patient's ventricular contractions (represented by the QRS complex) and only delivers an electrical stimulus (at a predetermined rate) if no contraction occurs.	Right ventricle
FIXED (example B)	Pacemaker senses the patient's ventricular contractions (the QRS complex) and fires continuously. If heart rate falls below a predetermined rate, this firing replaces the QRS complex. If the heart rate stays at or goes faster than a predetermined rate, the pacemaker keeps pace with the contractions, firing harmlessly into the patient's intrinsic QRS complex.	Right ventricle
DEMAND (example B)	Pacemaker senses atrial contractions, waits a predetermined interval, then fires into the ventricle. If no atrial contraction is present, the pacemaker fires into the atrium and the ventricle.	Right atrium and right ventricle

Advantages	Disadvantages	Effect on EKG waveform (S indicates pacemaker spike)
• Simple circuitry and mechanism	• Does not accommodate changes in patient's intrinsic heart rate • May cause cardiac arrhythmias • Atrium electrode placement will work only if the patient has an intact electrical conduction system	
• Accommodates changes in patient's intrinsic heart rate • Usually does not cause cardiac arrhythmias • Since pacemaker fires only when needed, battery often lasts longer than with fixed mode	• Complicated circuitry and mechanism	
• Accommodates changes in patient's intrinsic heart rate • Usually does not cause cardiac arrhythmias	• Complicated circuitry and mechanism	
• Accommodates changes in patient's intrinsic heart rate • Usually does not cause cardiac arrhythmias	• Complicated circuitry and mechanism	

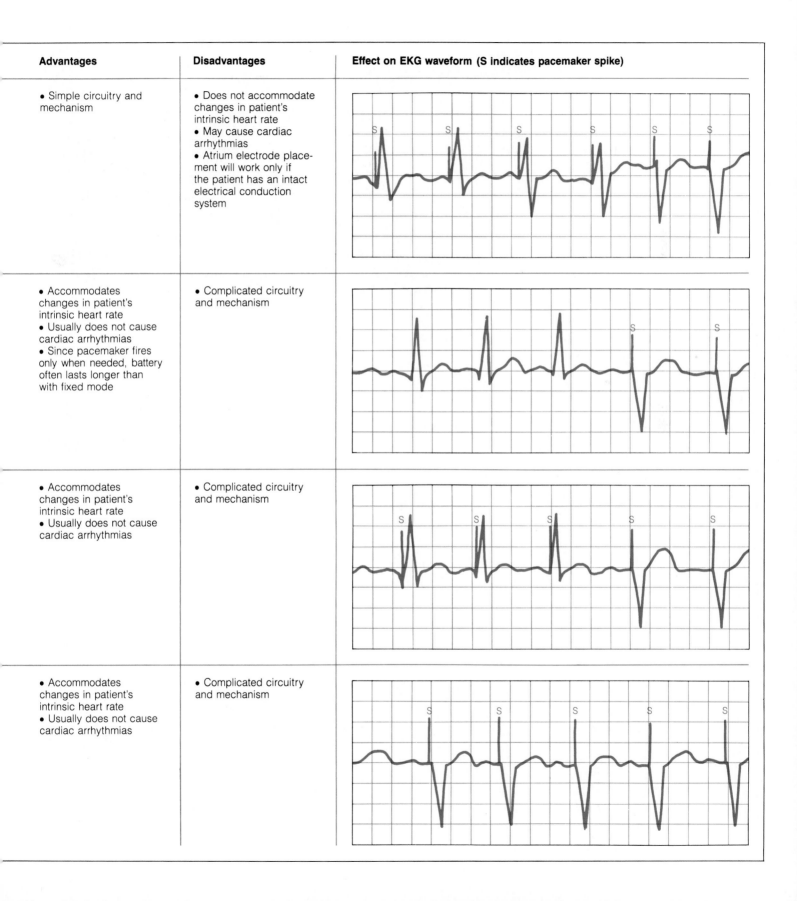

Cardiac pacemakers

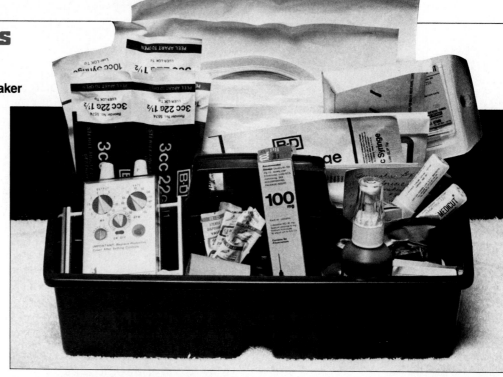

Helping to insert a temporary pacemaker

1 *Your patient, 29-year-old Sally Druzic, has been brought to the ED with a severe cardiac arrhythmia resulting from a Mellaril overdose. The doctor decides to insert a temporary pacemaker. He can insert the temporary pacemaker electrode into any of the following veins: subclavian, femoral, jugular, or basilic. (He also can insert it transthoracically, but doing so is hazardous and is attempted only in emergencies.)*

Suppose he chooses the subclavian vein. While he prepares for surgery, gather this equipment: skin prep supplies, sterile gloves, sterile towels, lidocaine 1% or 2%, a 5 cc syringe and needle, introducer wire, a sterile suture tray, antiseptic ointment, sterile gauze dressing, nonallergenic tape, and a temporary pacer and electrode.

2 Place the patient flat on her back. Prep the subclavian vein area of her chest and drape it with sterile towels, leaving a 4″x4″ (10x10 cm) area exposed.

The doctor will anesthetize the site and perform venipuncture with an introducer wire. After he enters the vein, he'll pass the electrode through the introducer. With guidance from fluoroscopy or an EKG, the doctor then advances the electrode into the heart's right ventricle.

Note: If an EKG is used, be certain it's battery powered or electrically approved for this procedure, to avoid the risk of electrical shock.

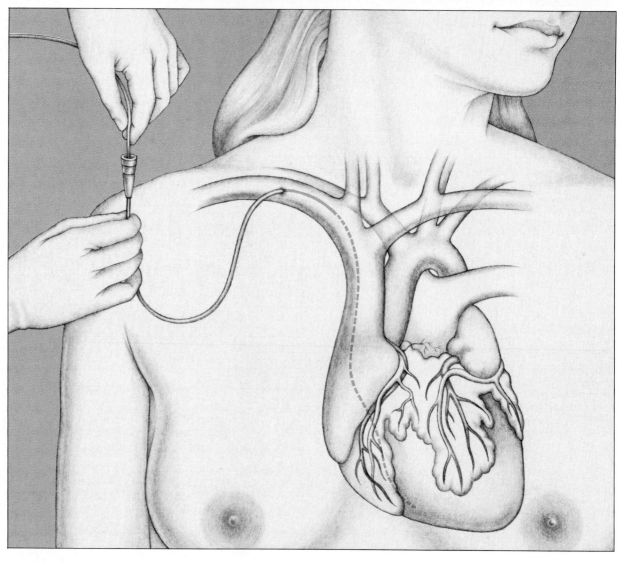

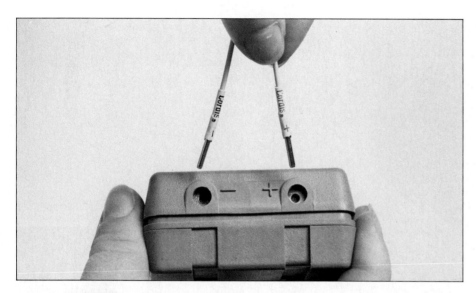

3 When insertion's completed, the doctor will check to make sure the temporary pacer's off. Then he'll connect the electrode wires to the two terminals on the pacer, with the positive or proximal wire matched with the positive terminal and the negative or distal wire with the negative terminal.

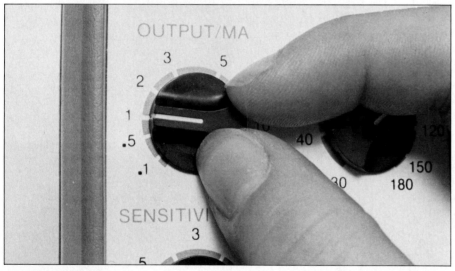

4 Set the pacemaker rate according to the doctor's orders. Set the milliamperes control at 1 MA, or as ordered, so the doctor can determine the cardiac threshold—which is the lowest level of electricity that can stimulate the patient's heart. When he has, he'll reset the millamperes at one and a half to two times the threshold. Then, turn on the pacemaker.

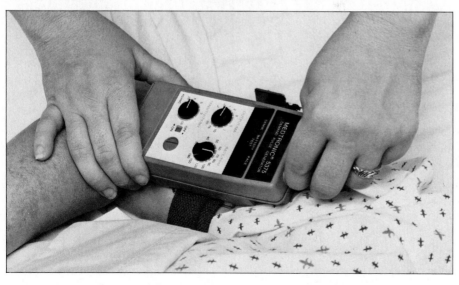

5 The doctor then sutures the electrode to the site and makes a stress loop of the remaining lead wire. Clean the area with alcohol and apply an antibiotic ointment. Cover the site with a sterile dressing and tape it. Secure the pacer to the patient's upper arm using the strap supplied by the manufacturer, as the nurse is doing here. If that's not available, use a Kling or Ace Bandage instead. Place the cap that's supplied by the manufacturer over the pacer controls. This way the settings can't be changed accidentally.

The doctor will confirm proper electrode placement with an X-ray or 12-lead EKG. Finally, document the following: type of pacer used, date of insertion, doctor's name, control settings, if the pacemaker successfully treated the patient's arrhythmias, and other pertinent observations.

Cardiac pacemakers

Helping to insert a permanent pacemaker

1 *If the doctor decides your patient needs a permanent pacemaker, you may be asked to assist with its insertion. Do you know how? This photostory shows you.*

Gather this equipment, taking care to observe aseptic technique: a cardiac pacer and electrodes, sutures, scalpel, lidocaine, 5 cc syringe and assorted gauge needles, povidine-iodine, sterile drape, nasal cannula, oxygen, sterile gauze dressing, alcohol swabs, antiseptic ointment, and nonallergenic tape.

The doctor will perform the procedure in an operating room, X-ray room, or cath lab.

Chances are, he'll insert the electrode in the subclavian vein (though insertion can also be done through the cephalic, femoral, jugular, or basilic vein). However, if the patient has arterial sclerosis or extremely weak cardiac tissue, the doctor may insert the electrode epicardially or by thoracotomy.

For the patient shown here, the doctor's chosen the subclavian vein.

Place the patient flat on his back. The doctor may ask you to insert a nasal cannula so he can deliver oxygen to the patient during the procedure. Make sure limb leads for a 12-lead EKG are in place and connected to a monitor that's battery powered or electrically approved for this procedure (to avoid shocks). Prep the insertion site and drape it with sterile towels, as ordered. In most cases the doctor will then inject a local anesthetic but he may use a general anesthetic.

2 The doctor then makes an incision in the patient's chest and nicks the subclavian vein. He'll pass the electrode into the right atrium or ventricle of the heart, aided by fluoroscopy.

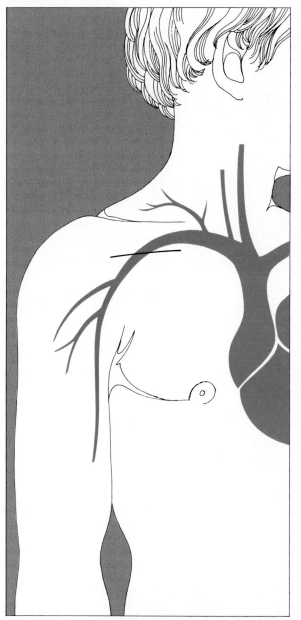

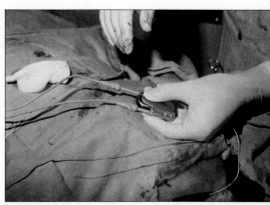

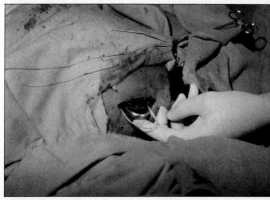

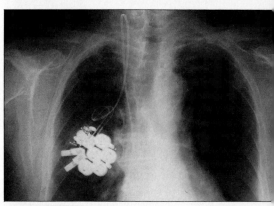

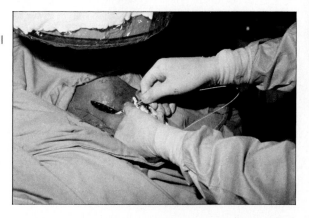

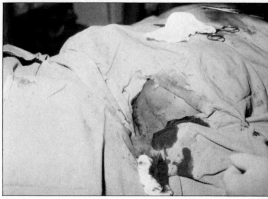

3 Then he'll individually test the electrical function of the electrode and the pacer. If the electrode fails to stimulate the heart sufficiently, he'll reposition it and test it again. If the pacer doesn't work, he'll replace it.

4 When he obtains good electrode placement, he'll create a pocket in the patient's chest (usually near the electrode insertion site) and insert the pacer into it.

5 The doctor may order an X-ray to confirm placement. This X-ray shows a permanent pacer positioned just below the right clavicle and an electrode placed in the right ventricle of the patient's heart.

6 After inserting the pacemaker, the doctor will close the incision with sutures. Then, he may ask you to clean the area with alcohol. After that, apply antiseptic ointment and cover the site with a sterile dressing. Secure it with tape.

If the patient has a temporary pacemaker, the doctor will probably leave it in for 24 hours following the insertion, just in case the permanent pacemaker is not functioning properly.

Programming the permanent pacemaker

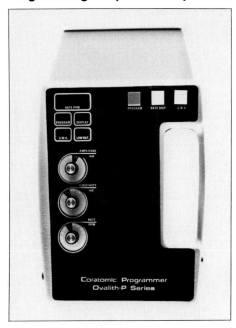

Coratomic Programmer
Ovalith-P Series

Your patient has a permanent pacemaker in his chest. When the pacemaker was inserted, it was set to stimulate the patient's heart if the patient's heart failed to beat at least 70 times a minute. Now, the doctor orders the beats per minute (BPM) level decreased to 60. Here's how it's done:

Many of the newer permanent pacemakers are constructed in such a way that the doctor can alter their settings noninvasively. All he needs is a special programmer, like the one shown here.

To use it, the doctor positions the head of the programmer no more than 3″ (7.5 cm) away from the area where the pacer is implanted. Then, by working the controls on the face of the programmer, he can send out electronic signals that change the pacemaker setting beneath the skin.

Note: The programming process is complicated and should never be attempted by untrained personnel.

Troubleshooting cardiac pacemakers

As you know, pacemakers can cease to function because of battery depletion. But random problems, such as those listed here, may occur at any time and cannot be predicted. Learn their cause and how to deal with them *before* they occur.

Pacemaker problem	Possible cause	Possible solution
Loss of capture (the inability to stimulate the heart)	• End of life or premature battery depletion • Lead wire fractured • Electrode tip out of position • Circuitry component failure • Cardiac perforation by electrode tip • Low capture threshold setting	• Doctor may replace battery. • Doctor may replace lead wire. • Turn patient onto his opposite side to reposition electrode tip. • Doctor will draw back slightly on the lead wire to reposition the electrode tip. • Doctor may have to replace pacemaker.
Heating up, reverting to an asynchronous mode, or changing program values (These problems occur only with programmable pacemakers.)	• Electromagnetic interference (EMI), from diathermy, power tools, appliances, or other electrical equipment • Circuitry component failure	• Doctor will reprogram pacemaker. • Doctor may have to replace battery.

Cardiac pacemakers

Dealing with cardiac complications

Do you know the possible complications facing a patient with a pacemaker? You should familiarize yourself with their signs so you'll be able to notify the doctor immediately if you detect any problems. Then he can order treatment.

Patient problem	Cause	Solution
Premature ventricular contractions, ventricular tachycardia, ventricular fibrillation	• Myocardium irritated during implant	• Doctor will order medication, such as lidocaine hydrochloride (Xylocaine*) to treat irritability.
Myocardial hemorrhage	• Electrode tip placed in the epicardium	• If cardiac tamponade has occurred, the doctor may perform an emergency pericardiocentesis.
Swelling, redness, drainage, and pain at insertion site	• Local or systemic infection	• Doctor will probably order antibiotics. May remove lead wire and insert it at new site.
Fluid accumulation, pacer migration, and/or pocket erosion (for permanent pacemaker only)	• Body rejection	• Doctor will withdraw fluid with a needle and syringe. May reposition pacer.
Muscle twitching at the pocket site (for permanent pacemakers only)	• Misplaced electrode tip	• Doctor will pull back slightly on lead wire to reposition electrode tip.
Rapid hiccuping	• Misplaced electrode tip stimulating diaphragm	• Doctor will pull back slightly on lead wire to reposition electrode tip.

*Available in both the United States and in Canada

Caring for the patient with a pacemaker

How do you care for the patient with a newly inserted pacemaker? That depends on the patient's physical condition and the way the pacemaker electrode was inserted in his heart. The doctor will instruct you in the special care your patient should receive. But here are several care basics to guide you:
• Place the patient on a hardwire (continuous) monitor for the entire time the pacemaker's in place. Check his rhythm hourly. If you observe ventricular ectopic beats that may mean the electrode tip is not positioned correctly, or is irritating the ventricle wall, notify the doctor.
• Change the dressings and apply antibiotic ointment every 24 hours, or as necessary, if the dressing becomes soiled or the site is exposed to air.
• Check the insertion site for signs of bleeding, infection, swelling, redness, or exudate. The doctor may order prophylactic antibiotics for up to 7 days following the insertion.
• Check vital signs and level of consciousness every hour the first 4 hours, every 4 hours for the next 48, and then once a shift. Confused, elderly patients with second degree heart block will not have an improved level of consciousness right away.
• Check the peripheral pulses distal to the insertion site for signs of thrombosis, following the same frequency pattern as for vital signs.
• Relieve patient's pain or discomfort with analgesics, as ordered.
• Auscultate lungs and heart every shift for signs of rales, decreased breath sounds, or friction rubs.
• Ask the patient if he has experienced shortness of breath, palpitations, or hiccups. Record your findings.
• If you must move a patient who has a temporary pacemaker, elevate the affected extremity. This will ensure adequate circulation and immobilize the extremity. Do not move the patient up in bed by pulling his affected axilla. This may cause pacemaker catheter displacement. Instead, use a drawsheet to reposition him. Make sure the pacer is secure and its cap is in place.
• Encourage the temporary pacemaker patient to engage in active range-of-motion exercises with his unaffected extremities. Teach him how to do passive range-of-motion exercises with his affected extremity.
• After 1 day, allow your patient to get up and sit in a chair. But, warn him not to lift his affected arm above shoulder level (or as advised by the doctor) for 1 month, until fibrous tissue has formed completely around the electrode tip.
• If a patient needs his temporary pacemaker for more than 5 to 7 days, or if any signs of infection appear, the doctor will probably remove and replace the catheter.
• Post information about the patient's pacemaker near the patient's bed. Record this information on his chart as well. Include the following: pacer model and serial number, date of implant, location of pacemaker lead, location of pacer (if permanent), and pacing rate. Record baseline data using a 12-lead EKG and a chest X-ray.

Teaching your patient about his pacemaker

You confront two challenges when you teach your patient about his cardiac pacemaker. The first is to gear the sessions to your patient's intellectual capacity and interest level. The second is to recognize and allay his fears. These fears can range from an obvious one of death if the pacemaker fails to a subtle one of altered body image.

Begin your first session by reviewing the facts contained in the heart and pacemaker booklets that you gave your patient before the insertion. As before, you may want to show him a heart model, pacer, and electrode to demonstrate what you're explaining.

Your patient's ID card

While he's in the hospital, your patient will probably be issued a temporary ID card, like the one printed below, stating that he has a pacemaker. Explain that he must carry the card with him at all times. He'll be sent a permanent ID card after he returns home. Also, provide him with the information he needs to order an ID bracelet, like the one below. Encourage him to buy one and wear it at all times.

Does your patient have a nuclear pacemaker? If he plans to travel abroad, he must inform the pacemaker manufacturer of his travel itinerary, means of travel, and the name of the doctor supervising his care. This is a requirement of the Nuclear Regulatory Commission.

Tell your patient that airport security systems will detect his pacemaker. To board the plane, he may have to show airline officials his ID card.

Teach your patient to take his pulse

After he's discharged from the hospital, your patient should take his pulse daily, preferably when he's sitting in a comfortable chair, or sitting up in bed. Make sure he obtains a *resting* pulse rate; for example, just before getting out of bed each morning. He should take his pulse for at least 1 minute. On teaching your patient how to take his pulse, turn to page 127.

For your patient to assess his pulse rate, he must understand his pacemaker mode. If the patient has a demand pacemaker, his intrinsic heart rate may be higher than the set rate of the pacemaker. This may cause him undue concern. Remind him that his pacemaker is an emergency backup system—for example, if his heart rate should decrease while he's asleep, the pacemaker will take over and maintain his heart rate at the predetermined level. Inform him of what pulse discrepancy is acceptable, what is not, and who to call when the discrepancy is unacceptable. Write down this information for him.

Pacemaker information

Supply the patient with information on the pacemaker's warranty and the life expectancy of the pacemaker battery (see the chart on page 107). If pertinent, alert him to the fact that if the battery runs down, the pacer may need to be replaced. If it does, he'll be hospitalized for a couple of days. To replace the pacer, the doctor will inject a local anesthetic and open up the scar. Next, he'll disconnect the lead wire and remove the old pacer. Then he'll insert a new pacer and reconnect the old lead wire. After the doctor closes the incision, the patient should be monitored for at least 24 hours, to make sure the new battery is working.

Limitations

Make the patient aware that he should approach electrical machinery with caution. In general, modern pacemakers have a shield to protect them from electromagnetic signals given off by machinery, but caution must always take precedence. If the patient feels lightheaded or uncomfortable near machinery, he should immediately back away until the feeling is gone. So he feels more secure, suggest that another person be nearby when he's dealing with a machine, especially for the first time.

Follow-up care

Follow-up care is part of every pacemaker patient's life whether he receives that care in a doctor's office or by transtelephonic monitoring. Here's how one type of transtelephonic monitoring works:

The patient is sent home with a small magnet that has an electrode clip attached to one end and a small wooden receptacle attached to the other end. The patient is given a time every month (or more often depending on his condition) to call a special number supplied by the manufacturer. When he makes the call, he'll be told to place the phone receiver into the wooden receptacle, the magnet over his pacer, and the clip on his index finger. This way, his EKG can be transmitted over the telephone.

The frequency of office visits or phone calls that the patient must make depends on the patient's needs and the power source used in his pacemaker. As his pacemaker gets older, his frequency of visits or phone calls will increase. He should expect this.

PACEMAKER IDENTIFICATION CARD

Name: _____
Address: _____
Phone: _____ Blood type: _____

I am wearing a pacemaker. In an emergency, contact:

Doctor: _____
Address: _____
Phone: _____
Date of implant: _____
Hospital: _____
Address: _____
Phone: _____

Type of pacemaker: _____
Manufacturer: _____
Paced rate: _____
Type of leads: _____
Model: _____
Serial number: _____

Please! Carry this card at all times.
It will help others assist you in an emergency.

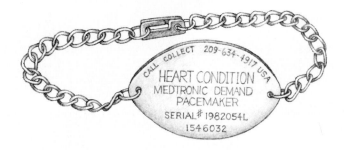

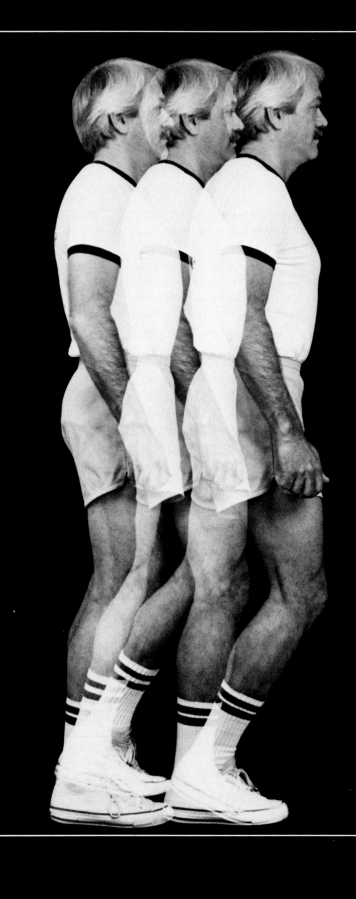

Rehabilitating Your Patient

Cardiac rehabilitation

Cardiac rehabilitation

A patient who's hospitalized with a cardiac condition may feel overwhelmed with despair. Chances are, he suspects that his best years are over. He worries that he'll never be able to resume all the activities he once enjoyed. In short, he feels that he's lost all control over his life.

Most likely, he's wrong. But, he'll need your help to understand why.

How can you help him? By implementing a comprehensive cardiac rehabilitation program that includes:
• teaching the patient about his condition and the lifestyle changes it requires.
• providing emotional and social support for the patient and his family.
• supervising a physical activity program.

In this chapter, we'll show you how to provide this help. Keep in mind that the specific programs we present are only examples—your hospital's program may be different in many ways. However, the goals are the same: to give your patient a sense of control over his life and health, and to encourage a positive approach to living with a heart condition.

Providing emotional support

Your hospital's chief administrator, Dr. Rosa Perez, was recently admitted to the ICU where you work. The admitting diagnosis: suspected inferior wall myocardial infarction (MI). Because she's a doctor, you expect her to be cooperative and knowledgeable about the care you give her. But to your surprise, she seems angry and resentful. "I've never been sick a day in my life," she complains to you. "Just because I'm under a lot of pressure doesn't mean I'm about to have a heart attack!"

Another patient in the ICU, Mr. Hearst, seems to be an entirely different type of patient. Also admitted with a suspected MI, Mr. Hearst is quiet and withdrawn. Although he's cooperative and easy to care for, you're concerned about his apparent depression.

Dr. Perez seems angry about her condition; Mr. Hearst seems depressed. Is either reaction unusual?

The answer is no. Nearly every patient with a serious cardiac condition initially experiences some emotional upset: panic, depression, sleeplessness, anxiety, anger. In fact, a cardiac patient probably feels *all* of these emotions, sooner or later.

And he's not alone. Almost certainly, his spouse and family feel upset too, although they may be reluctant to share their feelings with the patient.

How can you help your patient and his family understand these powerful emotions? Try planning several discussion sessions for the entire family. Your support and guidance can encourage them to cope realistically with their problems.

What you discuss in each session will vary. Be flexible—let

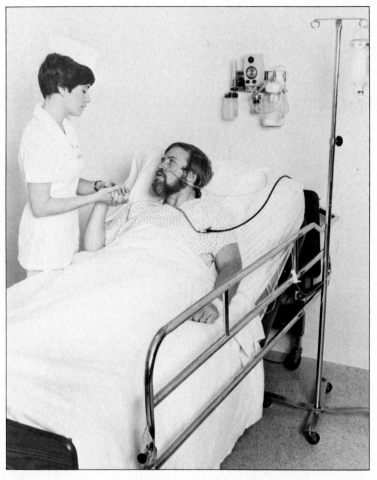

the patient and his family direct the discussions, according to their biggest concerns. But, use these suggestions as a guide:
• Explain common emotional responses evoked by an MI (and other acute cardiac events).
• Discuss the patient's personal reaction to his MI, and reassure him that his feelings are normal.
• Encourage the patient and his family to share their emotional reactions with each other.
• Discuss practical problems (medical expenses, for example), and refer the family to appropri-

ate agencies for help, if needed.
• Explain the lifestyle changes the patient faces after discharge, and suggest ways the family can adapt to them.
• Prepare the patient for feelings of depression and fatigue, which he may experience after he returns home.
• Recommend that the patient and his family join a support group, like the one shown on page 141. Such a group provides continuing support for the patient and his family throughout the recovery period.

Why exercise?

When your patient's recovering from an acute cardiac event, the doctor will prescribe a progressive activity and exercise program. How does such a program help your patient recover? As well as combating anxiety, fatigue, and depression, physical activity helps prevent or lessen these debilitating effects of prolonged bed rest:
• muscle atrophy
• orthostatic hypotension
• decreased lung volume

• decreased circulating blood volume
• moderate tachycardia in response to exercise
• negative nitrogen balance
• increased risk of thromboembolism.

Managing a 14-step rehabilitation program

Samuel Albin, a 60-year-old newspaper editor, has always led an active life. In addition to playing tennis several nights a week, he regularly hunts, fishes, and hikes on weekends. Now, he's in the hospital recovering from an anterior wall myocardial infarction, and he's not even allowed out of bed. Whenever he sees you, he peppers you with questions: "When can I get out of bed? Feed myself? Walk down the hall? Go home?"

Your answers depend on two things: first, the extent of damage to Mr. Albin's heart (the doctor determines this); and second, the type of inpatient physical rehabilitation program your hospital's developed. But one thing's certain. A gradual, but progressive, return to activity is just what Mr. Albin needs. Not only will it strengthen his heart, it'll reassure him that he can eventually return to an active life.

On the following pages, you'll see a 14-step inpatient rehabilitation program used at Albert Einstein Medical Center (Daroff Division) in Philadelphia, Pa. and developed at Grady Memorial Hospital, Atlanta, Ga. Your hospital's program may differ. For example, the exercises may not be the same. Or, the program itself may be shorter, to accommodate shorter hospital stays.

What are your responsibilities in carrying out a program such as this one? Once again, that depends on your hospital's policy. A physical therapist may supervise exercise activities while you supervise ordinary daily activities. Or, you may share responsibilities for both. (The doctor will determine how quickly the patient progresses from one step to the next.) Make sure you know exactly how your hospital's policy assigns responsibility.

Important: When you supervise your patient's physical rehabilitation, make sure he gets at least 1 hour's rest between daily activities and/or sets of exercises, unless the doctor directs otherwise. Remember, your goal is to exercise the patient's heart without overworking it.

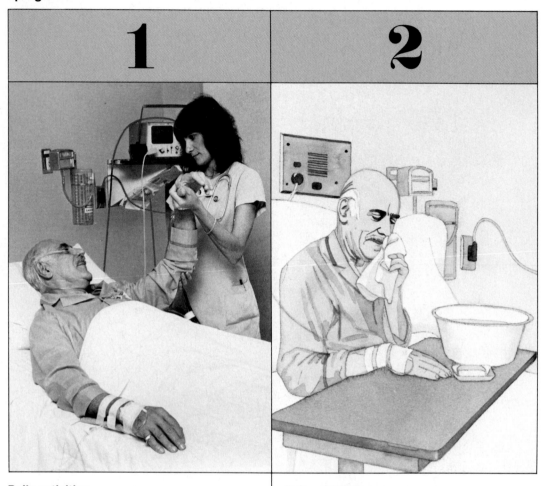

Daily activities
Tell the patient he must remain on bed rest, but also tell him he may:
• ask you to raise the head of his bed, if he wishes.
• feed himself in bed, with his trunk and arms supported.

Exercises
Perform the following passive range-of-motion (ROM) exercises for the patient, five times each, three times a day:
• shoulder and elbow flexion and extension
• hip and knee flexion and extension
• hip adduction and abduction
• foot rotation
• dorsiflexion and plantarflexion.

Daily activities
Tell the patient he may:
• wash his hands and face while remaining in bed.
• brush his teeth while remaining in bed.
• dangle his legs over the side of the bed once a day.
• use a commode for bowel movements.

Exercises
Continue to perform the passive ROM exercises listed in step 1, five times each, three times a day.

Cardiac rehabilitation

Managing a 14-step rehabilitation program continued

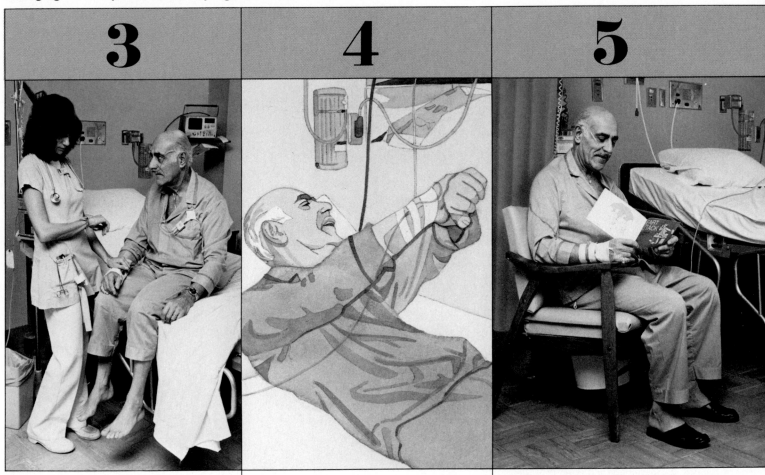

3

Daily activities
Tell the patient he may:
• wash his face, arms, and the front of his torso. (You'll wash his back and legs for him.)
• sit in a chair for 15 minutes, once a day.
• dangle his legs over the side of the bed one time a day.

Exercises
Ask the patient to perform ROM exercises himself, five times each, three times a day, while you support and assist him (active assistance ROM exercises). In addition, tell him to tighten the muscles in his legs and buttocks to the count of two. Conduct these exercises three times a day.

4

Daily activities
Tell the patient he may:
• wash himself and change his gown, with your assistance.
• use the commode whenever he wishes.
• sit up, as long as he's comfortable.

Exercises
Elevate the bed to a 45° angle and ask the patient to perform ROM exercises 10 times, three times a day, without your assistance (active exercise).

5

Daily activities
Tell the patient he may:
• sit up for eating and other daily activities. (But instruct him to lie down whenever he's tired.)

Exercises
Elevate the head of the bed to a 70° angle. Then, ask the patient to perform ROM exercises while you apply slight manual resistance to his movement. (Have him do the same exercises listed in step 1, except for dorsiflexion and plantarflexion.) Help him perform these exercises 10 times, three times a day. In addition:
• tell him to place each hand on its corresponding shoulder and do elbow circles.
• help him walk 25 feet in his room two to four times a day. Instruct him to walk slowly (10 to 12 steps every 15 seconds).

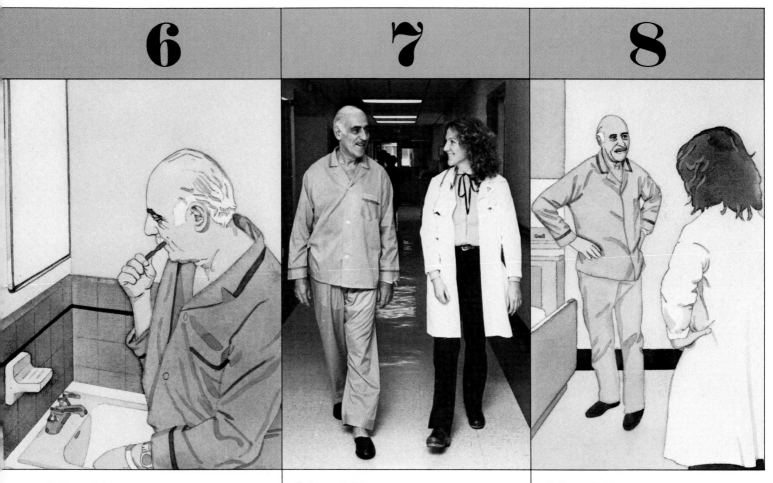

Daily activities
Tell the patient he may:
- wash himself at the sink.
- brush his teeth at the sink.
- use the bathroom in his room, or walk to the hall bathroom (if it's within 50 feet).
- go to the hall bathroom in a wheelchair (if the bathroom isn't within 50 feet).

Exercises
While the patient sits on the edge of his bed, apply moderate manual resistance as he performs the following ROM exercises:
- unilateral shoulder, knee, and hip flexion
- knee extension.
  In addition, accompany him on a 50-foot walk. Assist him, if necessary.

Daily activities
Tell the patient he may:
- walk to the hall bathroom.
- walk in the hall once a day, for a total of 75 feet.

Exercises
Teach the patient these standing warm-up exercises:
- arm rotations with hands on shoulders, arms abducted and elbows flexed. Repeat 10 times.
- raising body on toes with back pressed against a wall. Repeat 10 times.
- leg abduction and adduction.
  In addition, help him walk about 100 feet, with a rest stop.

Daily activities
Tell the patient he may:
- take a tub bath or sitting shower, with your supervision. *Important:* Make sure the water's warm, but *not* hot.
- use the bathroom, as needed.
- take two walks in the hall, 75 feet each time, at a speed of 10 to 12 steps each 15 seconds.

Exercises
Teach the patient these standing warm-up exercises:
- lateral side bending with hands on hips (five times for each side)
- trunk twisting, with hands on hips (five times for each side)
- slight knee bends (five times).
  Then, accompany him on a 150- to 200-foot walk, with a rest period. Later in the day, use a wheelchair to take him to a stairway. Help him walk down 2 flights of stairs (20 steps), with a rest every five steps. Make sure he rides the elevator back up. Push him in the wheelchair back to his room.

Cardiac rehabilitation

Managing a 14-step rehabilitation program continued

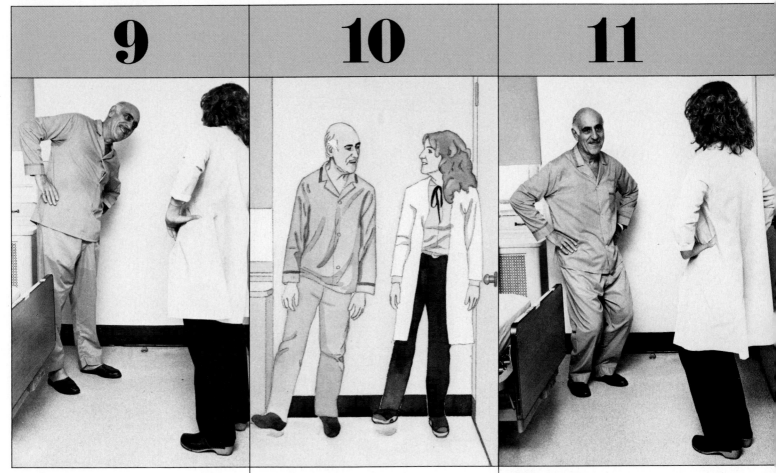

9

Daily activities
Tell the patient he may:
● walk, as desired.
● take a tub bath or sitting shower without your supervision. But, caution him not to use hot water.

Exercises
Supervise the warm-up exercises described in step 8. In addition, encourage him to walk at least 200 feet. Tell him to walk a little more quickly (15 steps every 15 seconds).

10

Daily activities:
Tell the patient he may:
● take a warm shower while standing, with your supervision.

Exercises
Supervise these warm-up exercises:
● lateral side bending, while you provide moderate manual resistance (five times each side)
● leg raising, with back against wall (five times each leg).
   In addition, encourage him to walk 300 feet. After a rest period, help him walk down 2 flights of stairs, with a rest between each five steps. Next, ask him to walk up and down two steps. Take the elevator back up.

11

Daily activities
Tell the patient he may:
● take a warm shower while standing, without your supervision.

Exercises
Supervise these warm-up exercises:
● lateral side bending, while you provide moderate manual resistance (five times each side)
● trunk twisting, with hands on hips (five times)
● leg raising, with back against the wall (five times each leg).
   In addition, encourage him to walk at least 300 feet. After a rest period, help him walk down 2 flights of stairs, resting between every five steps. Then, after another rest period, ask him to walk up and down four steps, two times. Using the elevator, take him back to his room.
   Note: The doctor may order a low-level treadmill exercise EKG for your patient. For details on supervising an exercise EKG, read pages 132 through 135.

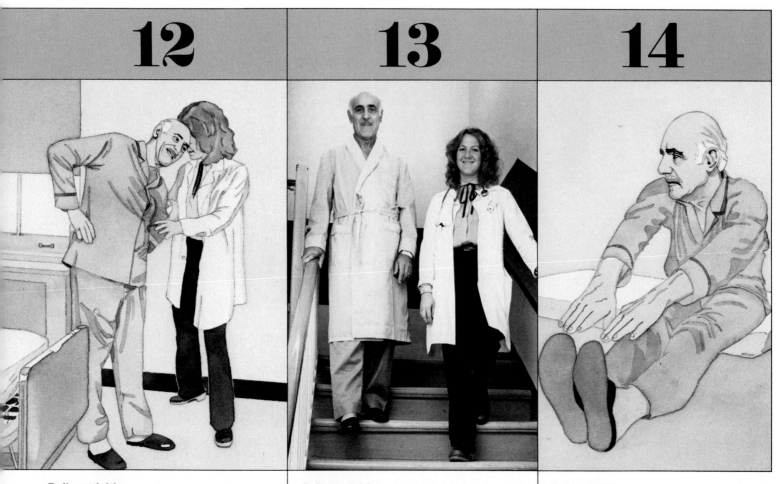

12

Daily activities
The patient may continue to engage in all the daily activities described in the preceding steps.

Exercises
Supervise the warm-up exercises listed in step 11, but instruct him to do each one 10 times.

Next, take him for a walk to a stairway; then walk down 2 flights of stairs, resting every five steps. Following a rest period, ask him to walk up and down 10 steps, resting every five steps. After he's rested again, encourage him to walk in the hallway at a speed of 15 steps each 15 seconds, for 2½ minutes.

13

Daily activities
The patient may continue to do all the daily activities described in the preceding steps.

Exercises
Repeat the warm-up exercises, as described in step 12. In addition, encourage the patient to walk in the hallway at a speed of 15 steps each 15 seconds, for five minutes.

When he's rested, ask him to walk up and down 10 steps, resting every five steps. After another rest, ask him to repeat this exercise.

14

Daily activities
The patient may continue to do all the daily activities described in the preceding steps.

Exercises
Supervise the patient in these warm-up exercises:
• lateral side bends and trunk twists, as described in step 12
• toe touches from a sitting position (10 times).

In addition, ask him to walk in the hallway for 5 minutes, at a slightly faster pace than described in step 13.

Ask him to walk down 2 flights of stairs (resting every five steps) and up and down 20 steps (resting every five steps).

Cardiac rehabilitation

Teaching your patient about heart disease

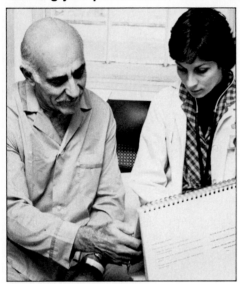

How can you educate your patient about his heart condition, and teach him to live with it? The chart below shows one teaching program. You may use this program (or one like it) in either group or individual teaching sessions.

Which type of teaching session is better? That depends. Group sessions have two advantages: they use your time efficiently, and they encourage support and sharing among group members.

But group sessions have one major disadvantage. They're not as effective as individual sessions for meeting each patient's special needs. As a result, you may prefer to teach some topics (risk-factor modification, for example, or returning to sexual activity) in individual sessions.

Use your judgment. Don't hesitate to teach your patient individually whenever it seems appropriate.

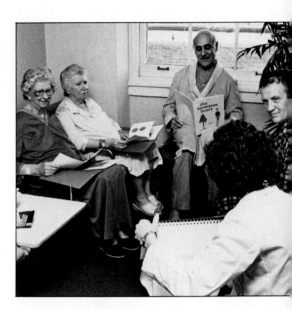

Cardiac teaching program: Five sessions

ONE	TWO	THREE	FOUR	FIVE
• How the heart functions (including its anatomy) • How and why the coronary arteries harden • How the heart heals after a heart attack • How the heart's affected by these risk factors: stress; smoking; high blood pressure; high cholesterol and triglyceride levels in blood; obesity; uncontrolled diabetes; lack of exercise; and family history	• What the patient's personal risk factors are • How to reduce his risk factors while he's in the hospital • How to minimize his risk factors after discharge	• How blood cholesterol contributes to hardening of the coronary arteries • How the patient can reduce the level of blood cholesterol by limiting saturated fats in his diet • How excess sodium contributes to fluid retention • What foods and seasonings contribute to excess sodium • How to recognize the warning signs of fluid retention • How excess weight contributes to heart disease • How to devise a plan for losing excess weight	• How a progressive activity program helps the heart heal • What activities are appropriate for the patient after discharge • When the patient may resume sexual activity, and what precautions to take (see page 127) • How to devise a plan for conserving his physical energy during usual daily activities • Why he should continue with an exercise program after discharge • How he should take his own pulse (see page 127)	• How to recognize signs and symptoms of heart attack, and distinguish them from those of angina pectoris • How to devise a plan for responding to a heart attack (or other cardiac emergency) • What medications the doctor's prescribed, and what each one's for • How and when to take each medication • What side effects are possible with each medication, and how to deal with them • What special precautions his medications require

Teaching your patient how to take his own pulse

When your patient begins an exercise program, his doctor will set progressive, target heart rates for him to achieve. For example, in the early phases of rehabilitation, the doctor may want him to exercise until his heart rate reaches 110 beats per minute. As rehabilitation advances, the doctor may want him to achieve progressively higher target heart rates.

To comply, the patient needs to know how to take his own pulse. Begin teaching him by explaining why he needs to monitor his heart rate during exercise. For example, say something like this: "Your heart's a muscle that needs exercise to stay in shape. That's why the doctor wants you to temporarily raise your heart rate slightly every few days. However, he doesn't want you to overwork your heart while it's still healing.

"To make sure you give your heart no more than the correct amount of work, you must know how to take your own pulse. The number of pulse beats you count each minute is the same as the number of times your heart beats every minute."

Next, make sure the patient understands the target heart rates his doctor's set for him. Explain that these target heart rates are based on the results of his exercise EKG. Then, answer the patient's questions.

Now, you're ready to show him the proper technique for taking a pulse. Make sure he has a watch or clock with a second hand. Then, show him how to place his index and middle fingers on his radial pulse. Warn him not to use his thumb. As you know, the thumb has a strong pulse of its own, which may confuse him.

Tell the patient to press firmly, until he feels the pulse beat. Ask him to count the beats for exactly one minute, while he observes his watch's second hand.

Important: To take his pulse rate during exercise, the patient should count for only 15 seconds, then multiply by four. He may cool down too quickly if he counts an entire minute.

For safety, do not encourage the patient to take his carotid pulse. Pressure on the carotid artery may produce arrhythmias or asystole.

Will the patient be exercising at home? Encourage him to write down his pulse rate, the time, date, and what he was doing just before taking his pulse. His doctor will use this information to assess the patient's recovery.

Important: Instruct the patient to call the doctor if his pulse ever seems faint, irregular, too fast, or too slow.

Counseling the cardiac patient about sex: What you should know

Thomas Cohn, a 62-year-old patient with a cardiac condition, is in a dilemma: He'd like to know if he can resume sexual activity with his wife—but he's too shy to ask anyone about it. Don't wait for Mr. Cohn to bring up the topic. Instead, take the initiative yourself.

How can you approach the subject without embarrassing Mr. Cohn? Try breaking the ice by giving him a book or pamphlet on sexual activity for patients who've had heart attacks. (See the books and pamphlets for patients listed on page 157.) Then, after he's done some reading, ask for his comments.

If Mr. Cohn refuses to discuss the subject, respect his wishes. But chances are, when he knows the subject's not taboo, he'll eagerly share his concerns.

What do you need to know in order to answer his questions? Read what follows:

Q. Is sexual activity dangerous for a cardiac patient?

A. No, provided the doctor's given him an OK. For the heart, sex is just a moderate form of exercise, no more stressful than a brisk walk. However, sexual activity can become dangerous if it's accompanied by great emotional stress. For example, the patient may place an additional burden on his heart if he has extramarital sex.

Q. When can my patient safely resume sexual activity?

A. That's up to the doctor, based on his assessment of the patient's recovery. But most patients can resume sexual activity within 6 weeks of a heart attack.

Q. Should my patient reduce or modify sexual activity?

A. Probably not, unless he suffers from advanced congestive heart failure, unstable arrhythmias or angina, or severe heart tissue damage. If his sex life must be curtailed for one of these reasons, suggest that he and his partner receive special counseling from a sex therapist, marriage counselor, or psychiatrist.

Q. Should my patient take any special precautions during sexual activity?

A. Yes. For guidelines, review the list of Do's and Don'ts below.

Q. How can I help if the patient loses sexual desire or his ability to perform?

A. Try to find the cause of the problem. Some patients lose their desire for sex because they're depressed. Others are afraid sex will trigger another heart attack. (The partners of cardiac patients may be overcome by this fear, too.) If your patient's fearful or depressed, urge him to discuss his anxieties with his partner. Counseling, education, and support by you, or a professional therapist or support group will also help.

Keep in mind that cardiac medications may cause impotence in some patients. If your patient suffers this side effect, tell him to discuss it with his doctor.

Resuming sexual activity: What the patient should know

Don't let your patient leave the hospital before you've discussed how he can safely resume sexual activity. If possible, include his partner in the discussion. Use these Do's and Don'ts as a guide:

DON'T be afraid to resume sexual activity with your partner. A satisfying sex life can help speed your recovery.

DO choose a quiet, familiar setting for sex. A strange environment may cause stress. Make sure the room temperature's moderate; excessive heat or cold makes your heart work harder.

DO choose times when you're rested and relaxed. Avoid sex when you're fatigued or emotionally upset. A good time for sex is the morning, after a good night's sleep.

DON'T have sex after drinking a lot of alcohol. Alcohol expands your blood vessels, which makes the heart work harder.

DO choose positions that are relaxing and permit unrestricted breathing. Any position that's comfortable for you is OK. Don't be afraid to experiment! At first, you may be more comfortable if your partner assumes a dominant role.

DO ask your doctor if you should take nitroglycerin before sexual activity. This medication can prevent angina attacks during or after sex.

DO call your doctor at once if you have any of these symptoms after sexual activity:
- sweating or palpitations for 15 minutes or longer
- breathlessness or increased heart rate for 15 minutes or longer
- chest pain or angina that's not relieved by two or three nitroglycerin tablets and/or a rest period
- sleeplessness after sexual activity, or extreme fatigue the following day.

Cardiac rehabilitation

Holter monitoring: The hows and whys

Holter monitoring provides a record of how your patient's heart functions over a 24-hour period. Here's how it works: You'll apply electrodes to the patient's chest and show him how to wear a portable monitor around his waist or on his shoulder. As the patient goes about his normal daily activities, he'll record, in a diary, his activities and his feelings. At the same time, the monitor will continuously record his heartbeat. At the end of the 24-hour period, the patient will return the monitor and his diary to you.

Why is Holter monitoring so valuable? Because it helps the doctor to:
• identify and document cardiac arrhythmias associated with normal activity.
• correlate these arrhythmias with symptoms, such as syncope, palpitations, chest pain, light-headedness, or dyspnea.
• assess the effectiveness of antiarrhythmic drugs.
• monitor artificial pacemaker function.

Using a Holter monitor

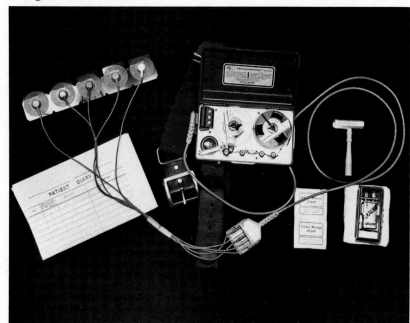

1 Edward Holand's recovering from myocardial infarction. To control dangerous cardiac arrhythmias, his doctor's prescribed procainamide hydrochloride (Pronestyl*). How well is this drug controlling Mr. Holand's arrhythmias? To find out, his doctor's ordered Holter monitoring. To prepare Mr. Holand properly, follow these steps:

First, gather the equipment shown here: a Holter monitor with tape reels and battery, a belted carrying case, skin electrodes (three for a single-channel monitor; four or five for a dual-channel monitor), 4"x4" gauze pads, alcohol swabs, razor and blade, nonallergenic tape (not shown), and patient diary.

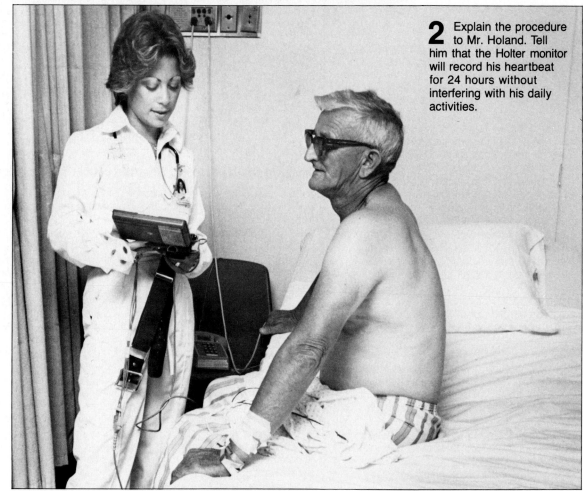

2 Explain the procedure to Mr. Holand. Tell him that the Holter monitor will record his heartbeat for 24 hours without interfering with his daily activities.

*Available in both the United States and in Canada

3 Now, get ready to prepare Mr. Holand's skin for electrode placement. In this photostory, we're featuring a dual-channel monitor that uses five electrodes. You'll apply them to the locations illustrated here. If your patient's chest is hairy, inform him that you must shave the hair at these locations.

Note: You may place the *ground* electrode anywhere on his chest.

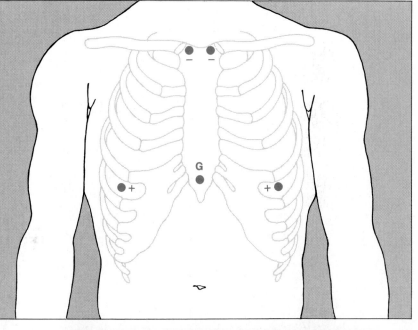

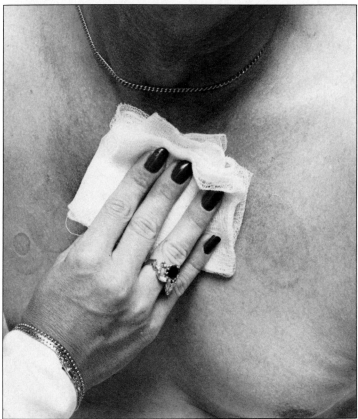

4 Use an alcohol swab to clean Mr. Holand's skin at one of these locations, and let the skin dry. (You'll get best results using a 99% alcohol swab.)

Then, slightly abrade the skin with a 4"x4" gauze pad, until you cause a red flush.

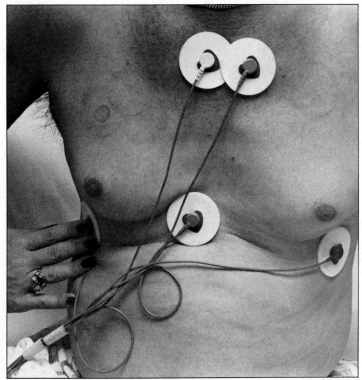

5 Peel off one electrode's backing and apply the electrode to the skin. Repeat this procedure until you've applied all five electrodes.

Then, ask Mr. Holand to hold the monitor and belt while you attach lead wires to the electrodes. (Not sure how to attach the lead wires? See page 76 for guidelines.)

Nursing tip: For added security, place a strip of nonallergenic tape over each lead wire.

Cardiac rehabilitation

Using a Holter monitor continued

6 Help Mr. Holand into his hospital gown. Then, turn on the monitor and place it securely in its case. *Note:* Some Holter monitors require calibration or the setting of a time clock before use. Does yours? Check the operator's manual for instructions.

Strap the case around Mr. Holand's waist, as shown here. Mr. Holand will be more comfortable if you strap it over his gown, instead of directly against his skin. Adjust the belt so it's comfortable, but don't leave it so loose that the monitor's weight strains the lead wires.

7 Now, explain to Mr. Holand that the success of this test depends on his cooperation. Show him the patient diary, and encourage him to record his activities and symptoms carefully. Give him a sample diary. If the monitor features an EVENT button, instruct him to press it if he experiences any unusual feelings.

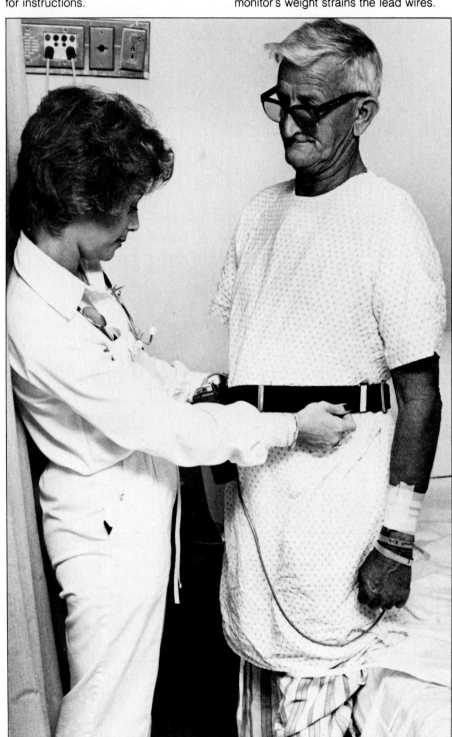

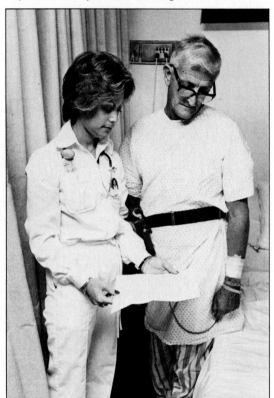

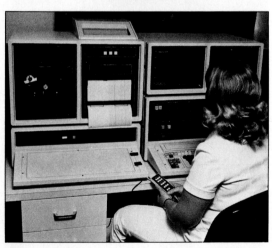

8 In 24 hours, remove Mr. Holand's Holter monitor and take his completed diary. A technician will use a computer, like the one shown here, to analyze the monitor's tape. Then, a cardiologist will compare the computer findings with the diary and interpret the results.

Patient teaching

Home care

What you should know about Holter monitoring

Dear Patient:
A nurse or cardiac technician has equipped you with a Holter monitor. Your doctor wants you to wear it to record your heartbeat over the next 24 hours. The information he'll gather from this recording will help him learn how your heart reacts throughout the day and night.

The success of this monitoring depends on your cooperation. For example, while you're wearing the monitor, the doctor wants you to write your activities and symptoms in a patient diary. Keep the diary and a pen or pencil with you at all times. Jot down the time of day you do any activity, such as the following: take medication (including nonprescription drugs), eat, drink (especially alcoholic or caffeinic beverages), move your bowels, urinate, engage in sexual activity, experience any strong emotion, exercise, or sleep.

Also jot down the exact time you had any physical symptoms; for example, dizziness, headache, pain, or shortness of breath.

Below is a sample of one patient's diary. Use it as a guide to help you complete your own diary.

Keep these additional guidelines in mind:
• Don't take the monitor out of its carrying case or meddle with it in any way. Do not disconnect the lead wires or electrodes on your chest.
• Don't let the monitor get wet. Don't shower, bathe, or swim with it on.
• Protect the cable and electrodes by wearing a T-shirt, especially while sleeping. (A woman may prefer wearing a nightgown.)
• Don't use an electric blanket during the monitoring period.
• Avoid high-voltage areas, magnets, and X-rays (including those used in airports).
• When the 24-hour period is over, return to the hospital with the monitor, and the nurse or technician will remove it. Do not remove it yourself.

Here are some extra instructions pertaining to your specific monitor:
_____
_____
_____
_____

TIME	ACTIVITY	SYMPTOMS
10:00 AM	Rode from hospital in car	Legs tired, some shortness of breath
11:00 AM	Watched TV in living room	Comfortable
12:15 PM	Ate lunch, took Inderal	Some indigestion
1:30 PM	Walked next door to see neighbor	Some shortness of breath
2:45 PM	Walked home	Very tired, legs hurt
3:00 4:00 PM	Urinated — Took nap	None
5:30 PM	Ate dinner, slowly	None
7:20 PM	Had bowel movement	Some shortness of breath
9:00 PM	Watched TV	Heart beating fast for about one minute, no pain
11:00 PM	Took Inderal, urinated, and went to bed	Tired
8:15 AM	Awoke, urinated, washed	Very tired, rapid heartbeat for about 30 seconds
10:30 AM	Returned to hospital	None, felt better

Cardiac rehabilitation

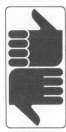

Is an exercise EKG indicated?

The doctor may order an exercise EKG (stress test) to:
• assess the patient's tolerance for exercise after a myocardial infarction or heart surgery.
• evaluate the patient's tolerance for increased exercise or activity.
• determine the effect of exercise on the occurrence of chest pain and other cardiovascular symptoms.
• identify arrhythmias caused by exercise.
• assess the effect of antiarrhythmic medication during exercise.

But, because an exercise EKG places an additional burden on the heart, it may cause dangerous cardiac complications, such as a myocardial infarction. So, for the patient's safety, the doctor may *not* order an exercise EKG if the patient has one or more of these conditions:
• uncontrolled arrhythmias
• uncorrected disease of a heart valve
• ventricular or dissecting aortic aneurysm
• heart chamber enlargement (cardiomegaly)
• severe anemia
• myocarditis
• pericarditis
• unstable angina
• uncontrolled hypertension
• congestive heart failure.

Preparing the patient for an exercise EKG

Bob Gannon, a 33-year-old photographer, suffered an inferior wall myocardial infarction (MI) almost a year ago. He's recovered so well that he's eager to resume his favorite sport, distance running. To assess Mr. Gannon's tolerance for such strenuous exercise, his doctor's ordered an exercise EKG.

Because Mr. Gannon's general health is good, and because his resting 12-lead EKG is stable, the doctor's scheduled him for a progressive, multistage treadmill test called the Bruce test. As the chart on the opposite page shows, Mr. Gannon will begin walking on a slow-moving treadmill that's tilted upward at a 10% angle. *Note:* Your patient may perform a progressive, multistage exercise test on a bicycle instead of a treadmill.

As the test progresses, the doctor increases the treadmill's speed and angle every 3 minutes. Before long, Mr. Gannon will feel like he's walking quickly up a steep grade.

As Mr. Gannon works, the doctor continuously monitors his heart with an EKG. In addition, he'll check his blood pressure at each stage.

What's the goal? To raise Mr. Gannon's heart rate to 173 beats per minute (bpm), or 90% of its estimated maximum ability. The doctor decides upon this heart rate by consulting a standard table, such as the one on the opposite page. Of course, if Mr. Gannon develops an unstable EKG or any of the danger signs listed on the opposite page, the doctor will stop the test before this heart rate's reached.

Note: The target heart rate that the doctor chooses depends on a patient's condition. For example, if the patient's elderly and has emphysema, the doctor will choose a much lower target heart rate.

Patient preparation

To prepare the patient for the procedure, the doctor takes a complete medical history and does a physical examination. In addition, he'll run a 12-lead EKG, to provide him with a baseline resting EKG. By comparing this to the exercise EKG, the doctor can see how the patient's heart responds to exercise. The doctor will also explain the procedure's risks, and ask Mr. Gannon to sign a consent form.

What's *your* role? At least a day before the test, give Mr. Gannon these preliminary instructions:

DON'T engage in strenuous activity for 12 hours before the test.

DO get a good night's sleep beforehand, and come to the test fresh and rested.

DON'T eat for at least 3 hours before the test. A full stomach competes with your heart for blood supply.

DON'T drink any alcohol, or beverages containing caffeine (such as coffee, tea, or cola) for at least 2 hours before the test.

DON'T smoke for at least 2 hours before the test.

DO wear loose, comfortable, cotton clothing: shorts or slacks, socks, and rubber-soled shoes such as sneakers. A woman should wear a bra, and a short-sleeved blouse that buttons in front. This way, the doctor or nurse can measure blood pressure, apply chest electrodes, and listen to her heart without removing her blouse. She shouldn't wear pantyhose. *Note:* Inpatients may wear pajamas.

DO continue to take medications as usual, unless the doctor directs otherwise.

Next, make sure Mr. Gannon knows what to expect. Describe the treadmill's operation to him, and explain that he'll work hard and become sweaty. Tell him he'll feel fatigued and slightly breathless, and encourage him to report his feelings to the doctor. Explain that you and the doctor will closely monitor his heart rate and blood pressure throughout the test. If necessary, explain how an EKG works. Finally, assure Mr. Gannon that he may stop the test whenever he wishes.

When you've explained the procedure to Mr. Gannon and answered his questions, he's ready for his exercise EKG the following day. In the next photostory, you'll see how to help supervise the procedure.

Important: Before conducting any exercise EKG, make sure the exercise room contains emergency medication and equipment, including: defibrillator, oxygen, airways, laryngoscope, syringes, needles, and I.V. setups. In addition, see that the room contains a chair, and a table or bed for the patient to lie on, if necessary.

The Bruce treadmill test: How it progresses

Stage	Speed (mph)	Speed (km/hr)	Grade (%)	Duration (minutes)
1	1.7	2.7	10	3
2	2.5	4	12	3
3	3.4	5.5	14	3
4	4.2	6.8	16	3
5	5.0	8	18	3
6	5.5	8.9	20	3
7	6.0	9.7	22	3

Determining a target heart rate

Age (years)	90% of maximum heart rate (beats per minute)
20-24	177
25-29	175
30-34	173
35-39	172
40-44	170
45-49	168
50-54	166
55-59	164
60-64	162
65-69	160
70-74	158

How to avoid overworking your patient

Your patient's undergoing an exercise EKG (stress test) on a treadmill. How much work can he safely do? You don't know for sure—after all, that's what the stress test helps you determine. So, to guard against the possibility of triggering a cardiac event during the test, you must closely monitor your patient's vital signs, and his heart rhythm and rate.

When do you know he's had enough? Criteria for stopping the test vary somewhat from hospital to hospital. (Make sure you know exactly what your hospital's policy requires.) Of course, you stop the test if your patient reaches the predetermined target heart rate. But, consider any of these danger signs reason to stop the test immediately:
• any decrease in systolic blood pressure below the patient's baseline resting level
• a decrease in heart rate that's 10 beats per minute below the patient's baseline resting level
• ST segment depression that's more than 2 mm below the patient's baseline resting level
• ventricular tachycardia (three or more consecutive PVCs), or frequent PVCs (five or more per minute)
• significant arrhythmias not present at rest
• chest pain not present at rest, or chest pain more severe than the patient would normally tolerate without taking nitroglycerin
• shortness of breath not present at rest
• diaphoresis or clammy skin
• dizziness, confusion, pallor, exhaustion, and/or claudication (staggering or ataxic gait)
• patient's request to stop the test.

Cardiac rehabilitation

Supervising an exercise EKG

1 *Your patient, Bob Gannon, has arrived at your outpatient facility prepared to take an exercise EKG. In response to your questions, he says he feels fine and is ready to begin. Here's how you help conduct the test.*

First, apply chest electrodes (following the procedure on page 73), according to the lead system selected by the doctor. If necessary, secure them with adhesive tape or a rubber belt.

Next, place the lead wire cable over the patient's shoulder and rest the lead wire box on his chest, as shown here. Secure the cable by taping it to his shoulder or back. Then, connect the lead wires to the chest electrodes. While you work, remind Mr. Gannon that you'll be monitoring his heart continuously throughout the test.

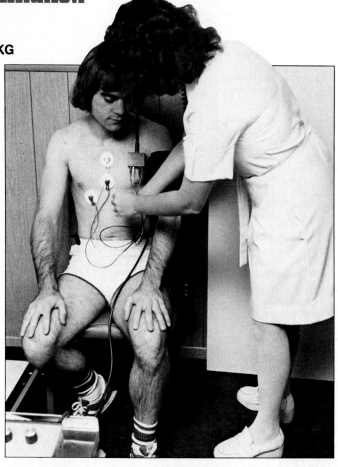

2 Now, while the patient's still sitting, take his blood pressure. This provides a baseline resting blood pressure. Document the reading.

Note: This patient's blood pressure cuff is connected to a special exercise test sphygmomanometer mounted on the wall.

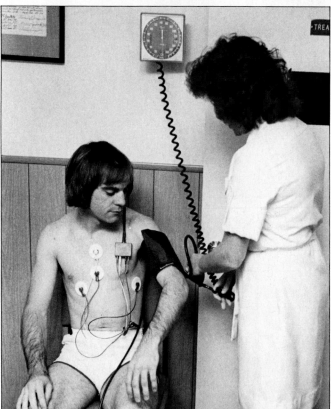

3 Next, turn the treadmill on to a slow speed, step onto it, and show the patient how to walk on it. As you do so, review some of the instructions you gave him earlier. For example, say something like this: "Begin walking very slowly, as I'm doing. While you walk, hold the bar lightly, without squeezing it. Use it for balance only. Don't look down. Look straight ahead, so you don't get dizzy.

"The doctor will slowly increase the speed and steepness of the treadmill. He'll alert you before each increase. By the way, don't be surprised if the treadmill makes a whining sound as it goes faster. As you work harder, we will see how your heart responds to exercise.

"Do as much as possible, but don't *overdo*. If you want to stop at any time, just tell us. Also, tell us if you feel dizzy, breathless, or tired out. We'll watch your blood pressure and EKG closely as you work."

4 Next, turn off the treadmill and ask the patient to step up on it. Before you turn on the treadmill, run resting EKG strips for the leads you plan to monitor during the test, and mark the strips, "Resting."

Then, you or the doctor should take another blood pressure reading. This provides a baseline resting blood pressure reading while the patient's in a standing position. Document the reading.

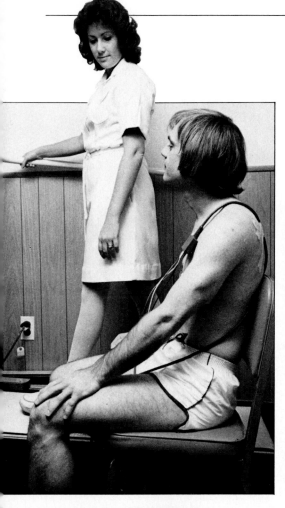

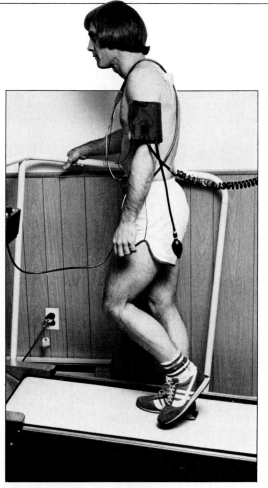

5 After alerting the patient, turn on the treadmill. As the patient walks, the doctor will monitor his heart, using one or more leads. He'll want you to periodically clip and mark portions of the strip for later analysis.

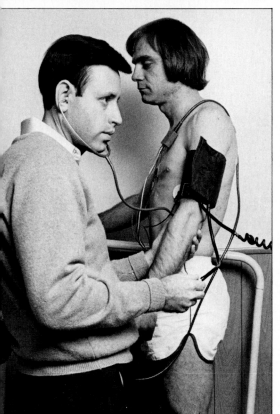

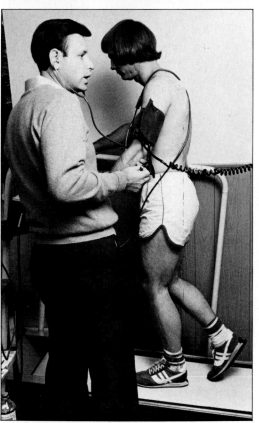

6 The doctor will periodically take blood pressure readings. Most likely, he'll take them at the end of each stage.

As the patient walks faster, don't forget to ask him how he feels. Is he tired? Does he have chest pain or muscle cramps? Is he out of breath? Does he want to stop the test? Remember, his feelings are just as important as his blood pressure readings and EKG tracings.

When Mr. Gannon reaches his targeted heart rate, or the doctor stops the test for any other reason, the doctor will slow the treadmill and tell the patient to continue walking for several minutes. This slowing-down period helps prevent the onset of dizziness or nausea.

Then, turn off the treadmill and help the patient to a chair. Continue to monitor his heart and blood pressure for 10 to 15 minutes, or until the EKG returns to the baseline reading.

Note: If the patient shows signs of discomfort at the end of the test, tell him to rest until these signs subside.

Remove the chest electrodes. Instruct the patient to wait at least 30 minutes to take a shower. Caution him to take a warm, not hot, shower. Hot water may cause him to faint or feel dizzy.

Cardiac rehabilitation

Using MET measurements to determine safe activity levels

After your patient's exercise EKG (stress test), the doctor tells you that the patient can safely tolerate 8 metabolic energy equivalents (METs) of activity. Do you know how this translates into daily activity? More important, can you explain it to your patient in words he'll understand? The information on this page can help.

A MET is an amount of metabolic energy your patient consumes at rest. When he uses 1 MET of energy, his body consumes about 3.5 ml of oxygen per kilogram of body weight each minute.

What does this mean to your patient? The chart below provides practical guidelines. Refer to it when you discuss safe activity levels with any patient. *Note:* Keep in mind that these are only general guidelines. General fitness, excitement, fatigue, or emotional stress may alter MET levels for any activity.

1 MET	1 to 2 METs	2 to 3 METs	3 to 4 METs	4 to 5 METs
Home activities • Bed rest • Sitting • Eating • Reading • Sewing • Watching television **Occupational activities** • No activity allowed **Exercise or sports activities** • No activity allowed	**Home activities** • Dressing • Shaving • Brushing teeth • Washing at sink • Making bed • Desk work • Driving car • Playing cards • Knitting **Occupational activities** • Typing (electric typewriter) **Exercise or sports activities** • Walking 1 mph (1.6 km/hr) on level ground	**Home activities** • Tub bathing • Cooking • Waxing floor • Riding power lawn mower • Playing piano **Occupational activities** • Driving small truck • Using hand tools • Typing (manual typewriter) • Repairing car **Exercise or sports activities** • Walking 2 mph (3.2 km/hr) on level ground • Bicycling 5 mph (8 km/hr) on level ground • Playing billiards • Fishing • Bowling • Golfing (with motor cart) • Operating motorboat • Horseback riding (at walk)	**Home activities** • General housework • Cleaning windows • Light gardening • Pushing light power mower • Sexual intercourse **Occupational activities** • Assembly-line work • Driving large truck • Bricklaying • Plastering **Exercise or sports activities** • Walking 3 mph (4.8 km/hr) • Bicycling 6 mph (9.7 km/hr) • Sailing • Golfing (pulling hand cart) • Pitching horseshoes • Archery • Badminton (doubles) • Horseback riding (at slow trot) • Fly-fishing	**Home activities** • Heavy housework • Heavy gardening • Home repairs, including painting and light carpentry • Raking leaves **Occupational activities** • Painting • Masonry • Paperhanging **Exercise or sports activities** • Calisthenics • Table tennis • Golfing (carrying bag) • Tennis (doubles) • Dancing • Slow swimming

5 to 6 METs	6 to 7 METs	7 to 8 METs	8 to 9 METs	10 or more METs
Home activities • Sawing softwood • Digging garden • Shoveling light loads **Occupational activities** • Using heavy tools • Lifting 50 pounds **Exercise or sports activities** • Walking 4 mph (6.4 km/hr) • Bicycling 10 mph (16.1 km/hr) • Skating • Fishing with waders • Hiking • Hunting • Square dancing • Horseback riding (at brisk trot)	**Home activities** • Shoveling snow • Splitting wood • Mowing lawn with hand mower **Occupational activities** • All activities listed previously **Exercise or sports activities** • Walking or jogging 5 mph (8.0 km/hr) • Bicycling 11 mph (17.7 km/hr) • Tennis (singles) • Waterskiing • Light downhill skiing	**Home activities** • Sawing hardwood **Occupational activities** • Digging ditches • Lifting 80 pounds • Moving heavy furniture **Exercise or sports activities** • Paddleball • Touch football • Swimming (backstroke) • Basketball • Ice hockey	**Home activities** • All activities listed previously **Occupational activities** • Lifting 100 pounds **Exercise or sports activities** • Running 5.5 mph (8.9 km/hr) • Bicycling 13 mph (20.9 km/hr) • Swimming (breaststroke) • Handball (noncompetitive) • Cross-country skiing • Fencing	**Home activities** • All activities listed previously **Occupational activities** • All activities listed previously **Exercise or sports activities** • Running 6 mph (9.7 km/hr) or faster • Handball (competitive) • Squash (competitive) • Gymnastics • Football (contact)

Save $2.00 off each NURSING PHOTOBOOK

Choose your first book. Examine it for 10 days FREE!

Subscribe to the NURSING PHOTOBOOK series and save $2.00 on every volume. That's a significant savings on the entire series. And now you can select your own introductory volume from the books shown or listed.

The NURSING PHOTOBOOK series

Aiding Ambulatory Patients • Assessing Your Patients • Attending Ob/Gyn Patients • Caring for Surgical Patients • Carrying Out Special Procedures • Controlling Infection • Coping with Neurologic Disorders • Dealing with Emergencies • Ensuring Intensive Care • Giving Cardiac Care • Giving Medications • Helping Geriatric Patients • Implementing Urologic Procedures • Managing I.V. Therapy • Nursing Pediatric Patients • Performing GI Procedures • Providing Early Mobility • Providing Respiratory Care • Using Monitors • Working with Orthopedic Patients

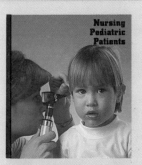

Nursing Pediatric Patients

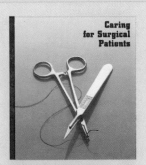

Caring for Surgical Patients

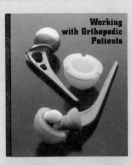

Working with Orthopedic Patients

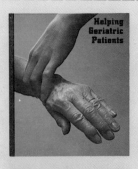

Helping Geriatric Patients

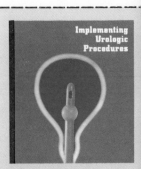

Implementing Urologic Procedures

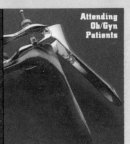

Attending Ob/Gyn Patients

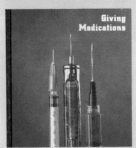

Giving Medications

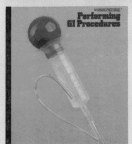

Performing GI Procedures

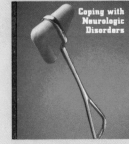

Coping with Neurologic Disorders

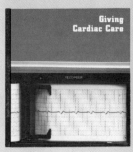

Giving Cardiac Care

© 1983 Intermed Communications, Inc.

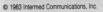

NEW!

FROM THE PUBLISHERS OF NURSING83® MAGAZINE.

Mail the postage-paid card at right. ▶

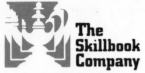
Introduce yourself to the popular NURSING PHOTOBOOK™ series

Each book in this unique series contains detailed *photostories*…and diagrams, charts, and anatomic illustrations to help you learn important new procedures. And each handsome PHOTOBOOK offers you ● 160 illustrated, fact-filled pages ● clear, close-up photographs ● convenient 9″ × 10½″ size ● durable, hardcover binding ● complete index. Watch the experts at work showing you how to… administer drugs…teach your patient about his illness and its treatment…minimize trauma… increase patient comfort…and more. Discover how you can become a better nurse by joining this exciting series. You can examine each PHOTOBOOK at your leisure… for 10 days *absolutely free!* Even if you've paid and later decide a PHOTOBOOK is not really helpful, you can return it at any time in the next 2 years, and we'll refund your money.

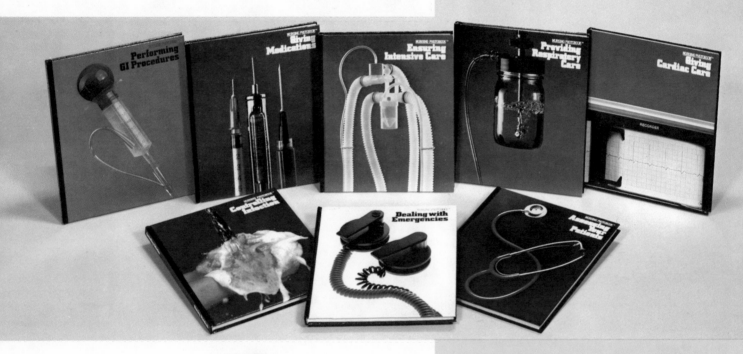

At last! A magazine that helps you with "the other side" of nursing. The things they didn't (and couldn't) teach you in nursing school.

NursingLife tells you how to be a better nurse…how to find greater fulfillment in your career…how to grow on the job.

It's about the *nonclinical* skills today's nurses need to round out their professional lives.

Become a Charter Subscriber to this exciting new magazine. Just tear off and mail this card today. There's no need to send money now. This is a no-obligation, free-trial offer!

If order card is missing, send your order to:

NursingLife®

P.O. Box 1961
One Health Care Circle
Marion, Ohio 43305

Combining an exercise EKG with perfusion imaging

Does your patient have coronary artery disease? To find out, the doctor may order perfusion imaging to accompany an exercise EKG.

Perfusion imaging is very similar to myocardial hot-spot imaging, which you learned about on page 57. But, instead of identifying *hot spots* in heart tissue, perfusion imaging identifies *cold spots*. Here's the difference:

For hot-spot imaging, the doctor or technician injects radioactive technetium pyrophosphate into the patient's bloodstream. Damaged heart tissue collects a large amount of this radioactive substance, which appears as a hot spot on film produced by a gamma scanner.

For perfusion imaging, the doctor injects a different radioactive substance, called thallium-201, into the bloodstream. This thallium, carried by the bloodstream, is distributed to the heart muscle. Poorly perfused tissue retains *less* thallium than adequately perfused tissue. As a result, poorly perfused tissue appears as a cold spot on film. Cold spots identify any tissue that's not supplied or is poorly supplied with blood; for example, newly infarcted tissue, scar tissue from old infarctions, or tissue that's supplied by an obstructed coronary artery.

Why combine perfusion imaging with an exercise EKG? Because perfusion imaging may identify ischemic areas that only appear when the heart's working hard and its need for blood increases. When the doctor sees how exercise affects the heart's blood supply, he has the information he needs to continue diagnostic studies or to prescribe a safe exercise program for the patient.

Preparing a patient for perfusion imaging with an exercise EKG

If your patient's scheduled for perfusion imaging along with his exercise EKG (stress test), prepare and care for him as you would for an exercise EKG alone (see page 132). But, in addition, tell the patient that the doctor's ordered perfusion imaging to accompany the exercise EKG, and explain why. Tell him that the doctor will insert a needle in a vein in his arm. Later, he'll use it to inject a small amount of radioactive thallium into the patient's bloodstream for the imaging. Assure the patient that the amount of radioactivity is very small—less than he'd receive from one X-ray. And remember to tell the patient that the procedure's painless (except for brief discomfort during needle insertion).

Note: An exercise EKG involves some risks, but perfusion imaging doesn't increase or compound the risks. After the doctor explains the risks to the patient, make sure the patient's signed a consent form.

Next, let your patient know what to expect during the procedure. Prepare him for all the strange equipment he'll see. In addition, describe the procedure itself, using these suggested comments as a guide:

• "After you've been exercising for a while, the doctor will inject thallium into a vein in your arm. Then, the doctor will ask you to continue exercising for several minutes."

• "Next, you'll be transported to the scanner room where the doctor will take pictures of your heart with a special scanner. These pictures will show how well your coronary arteries supply blood to your heart during exercise."

• "About 4 hours after you finish exercising, the doctor may take more pictures of your heart. They'll show him how well your coronary arteries supply blood to your heart after a rest period."

Note: The doctor may order perfusion imaging *without* an exercise EKG, to identify ischemic cardiac tissue that's present at rest. If he does, explain perfusion imaging to the patient. A perfusion test alone requires no special preparation, aside from the needle insertion. However, if your hospital requires it, make sure your patient's signed a consent form.

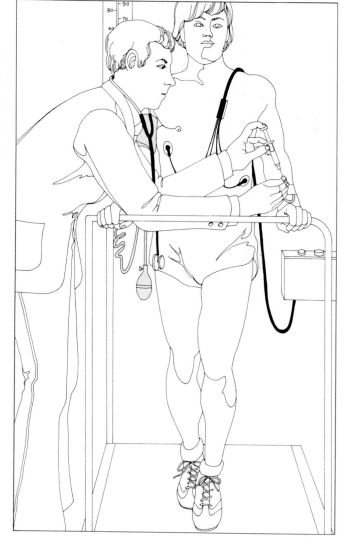

Cardiac rehabilitation

Establishing home exercise guidelines

Your patient's physical rehabilitation will continue after he leaves the hospital. Most likely, the doctor will prescribe an exercise routine that includes a daily walk. He'll also set a target heart rate for the patient to achieve.

Before the patient leaves your care, teach him how to determine his heart rate by taking his pulse (see page 127). Then, give him these exercise guidelines:
• Don't walk right after a meal. Wait about 2 hours.
• Don't walk in extreme heat or cold. The best temperature range is 40° to 85° F. (4° to 29° C.). If the weather's unpleasant, try walking in an indoor shopping mall.
• Wear comfortable shoes and loose-fitting clothes.
• Warm up for 3 to 5 minutes before walking (or beginning any other prolonged exercise). Perform the warm-up exercises you learned in the hospital or outpatient facility; for example, arm circles, toe raises, trunk twists, front and side bends, and stretching exercises.
• Walk at an even pace, maintaining the speed your doctor's prescribed. As you walk, rhythmically swing your arms at your sides.
• After your walk, cool down slowly. Walk in place while you take your pulse. Then, walk slowly for about 5 more minutes before stopping. This maintains good circulation while your heart rate returns to normal.
• Don't exceed your target heart rate. If your pulse rate rises above your target heart rate, walk more slowly next time.
• Notify your doctor if your pulse is irregular after your walk, or if you experience pain in your chest, teeth, ears, jaw, or arms; extreme breathlessness; extreme fatigue; dizziness, nausea, and/or vomiting.

Continuing rehabilitation after hospital discharge

Do you work in an outpatient cardiac rehabilitation facility? If you do, you're probably part of a team that includes nurses, doctors, and physical therapists. Together, you help patients return to active lives.

What's your role? In the next photostory, you'll see how to supervise an outpatient rehabilitation program. But because you're also responsible for tailoring the program to each patient's individual needs, you must assess the patient before he begins the program. To do this, follow these guidelines:
• Conduct a thorough assessment interview. Explore your patient's cardiac history, and note the medications he's taking. Then, find out how well he understands his condition, and identify his risk factors. Finally, try to determine how well he's adjusted, emotionally and psychologically, to his heart condition. All of this information helps you decide how much teaching and counseling the patient needs.
• Set rehabilitation goals, based on the patient's age, condition, and desired activity level. Discuss his plans with him. For example, let's say he plans to return to a job that requires lifting. In addition, he'd like to resume playing golf. To help him reach these goals, design an exercise program that emphasizes arm exercises, using equipment such as the rowing machine and arm ergometer.
• Obtain the results of a low-level exercise EKG (stress test). Most likely, the patient underwent this test before discharge. If not, the doctor will order one before the patient begins an exercise program. The information provided by an exercise EKG helps you and the doctor devise an appropriate exercise prescription for the patient.
• If ordered, take blood samples for laboratory studies. Once you know the fasting cholesterol, triglyceride, and high-density lipoprotein (HDL) levels of your patient, you can suggest diet modifications, if necessary.

When your assessment's complete, you can help the doctor design a rehabilitation routine that suits the patient. Read the photostory starting on the opposite page to learn how to implement it.

Learning walking speeds

When the doctor or physical therapist designs an exercise program for your patient, he'll specify walking speeds. For example, he may tell the patient to walk ¼ mile at a speed of 2 miles per hour (0.4 km at 3 km/hr). Can you explain to your patient what this means, in terms he can understand? Can you tell him how many metabolic energy measurements (METS) he consumes at each speed? Use this chart as a guide.

Speed mph	km/hr	Number of paces per second	Number of paces every 15 seconds	Number of paces every minute	METS
2 mph	3.2 km/hr	1	15	60	2 to 3
2.5 mph	4 km/hr	1	18 to 19	75	2 to 3
3 mph	4.8 km/hr	1	22	88	3 to 4
3.5 mph	5.6 km/hr	1	26	104	4 to 5
4 mph	6.4 km/hr	2	30	120	5 to 6
4.5 mph	7.2 km/hr	2	34	135	5 to 6
5 mph	8 km/hr	2	37 to 38	150	6 to 7

Note: 10 city blocks approximates 1 mile (1.6 km).

Supervising an outpatient rehabilitation program

In this photostory, you'll see one outpatient rehabilitation program. Each patient works independently, at his or her own speed. Here's how to supervise a program like this:

When the patient arrives for an exercise session, give him an exercise data sheet. Make sure you've already filled in this information: his name, weight goal, medications, target heart rate, and exercise prescription for the day.

Instruct the patient to record his heart rate after each phase of exercise. Tell him to let you know if the rate falls short of or rises above his target heart rate. In addition, tell him to document the exercise equipment he uses, as well as the duration of each exercise he performs. *Important:* Encourage him to tell you how he feels before, during, and after exercise.

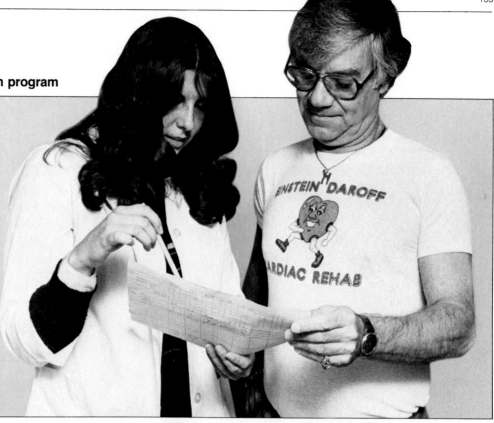

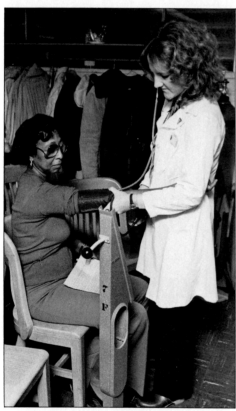

Take the patient's blood pressure and ask her to record it on the data sheet. This provides a resting baseline reading.

In addition, ask the patient to take her own pulse and record her heart rate on the data sheet.

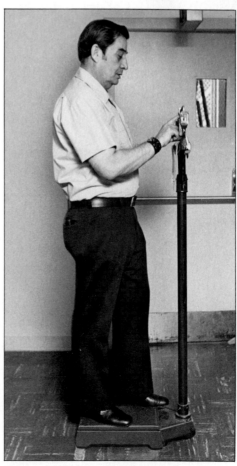

Next, the patient weighs himself, and records his weight on the data sheet.

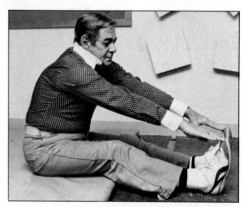

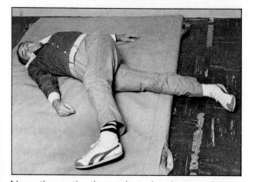

Now, the patient's ready to begin exercising, according to his exercise prescription. He'll begin with warm-up exercises, which gradually prepare his body for more strenuous work. Instruct the patient to warm up for about 10 minutes.

Explain how warm-up exercises help him avoid injuring his muscles and joints.

Cardiac rehabilitation

Supervising an outpatient rehabilitation program continued

Then, the patient can begin conditioning exercises. These exercises vary, according to the equipment available and the patient's exercise prescription.

Note: If your facility has an instant-EKG machine, spot-check the electrical activity of your patient's heart by running a rhythm strip at some time during the exercise routine. Mark the strip with the patient's name, the date, lead, and activity.

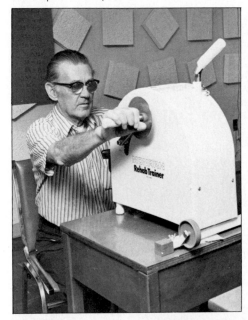
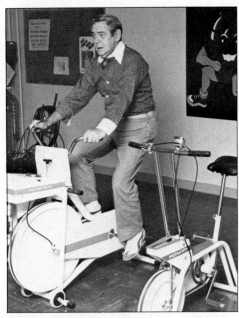

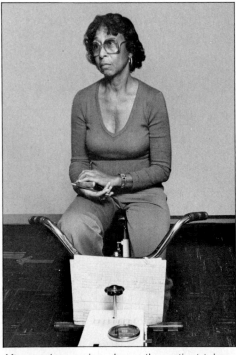

After each exercise phase, the patient takes her pulse and records it on her data sheet.

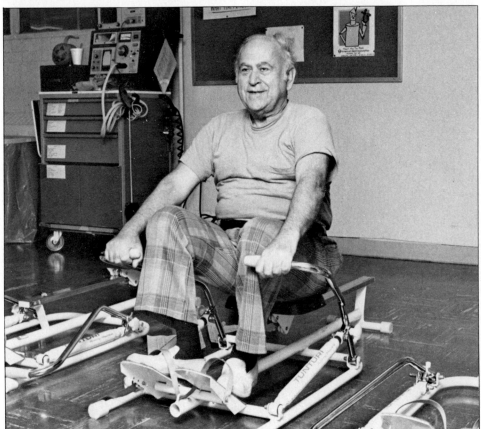

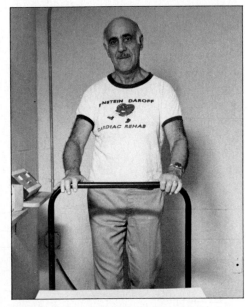

After exercise, the patient should cool down for about 10 minutes. This lets his heart rate and blood pressure decrease gradually, which prevents feelings of dizziness and nausea. This patient is cooling down by walking on a slow-moving treadmill.

Take the patient's blood pressure after he's cooled down. Then, make sure he records his blood pressure and post-exercise heart rate on the data sheet.

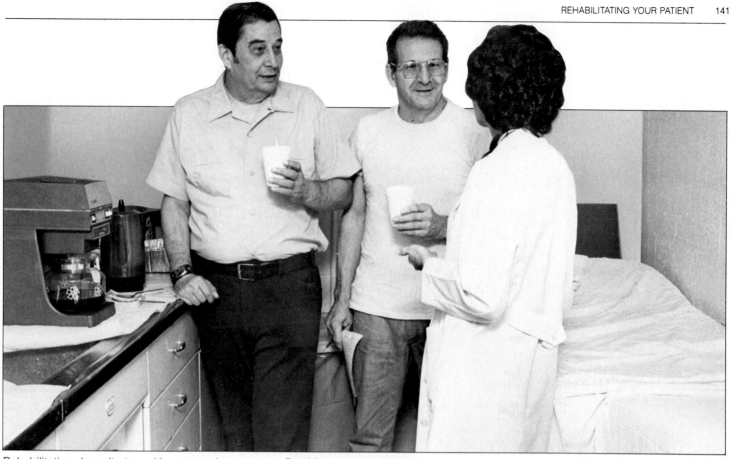

Rehabilitation doesn't stop with an exercise program. Provide support and education by joining informal discussions with small groups of patients. If they have any questions about heart disease, diet, risk factors, and exercise, answer them.

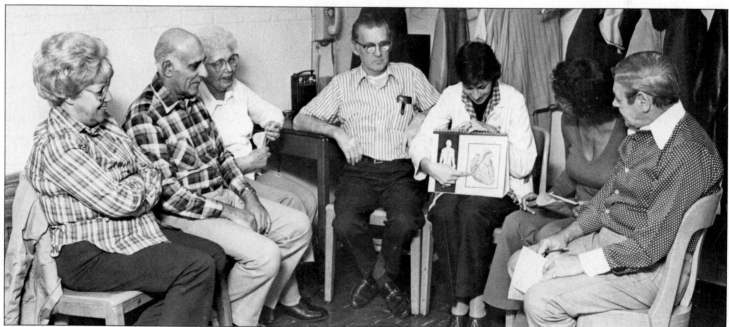

In addition, encourage each patient and his family to join a continuing education group. These groups allow you to continue teaching your patients how to live with heart disease. Group discussions, like the one shown here, also encourage sharing and emotional support among patients.

Note: Although most of your patients will return to active lives, some may face severe lifestyle changes. These patients need special counseling. Help them by organizing short-term group-therapy sessions supervised by a psychiatrist and a cardiac rehabilitation nurse. In addition, provide individual counseling.

After the patient's completed his rehabilitation program, encourage him to maintain a home exercise program. Teach him the home exercise guidelines on page 138. Then, check on his progress with weekly telephone calls. Finally, encourage him to stay in touch with his support group, and to return periodically for follow-up exercise test evaluations.

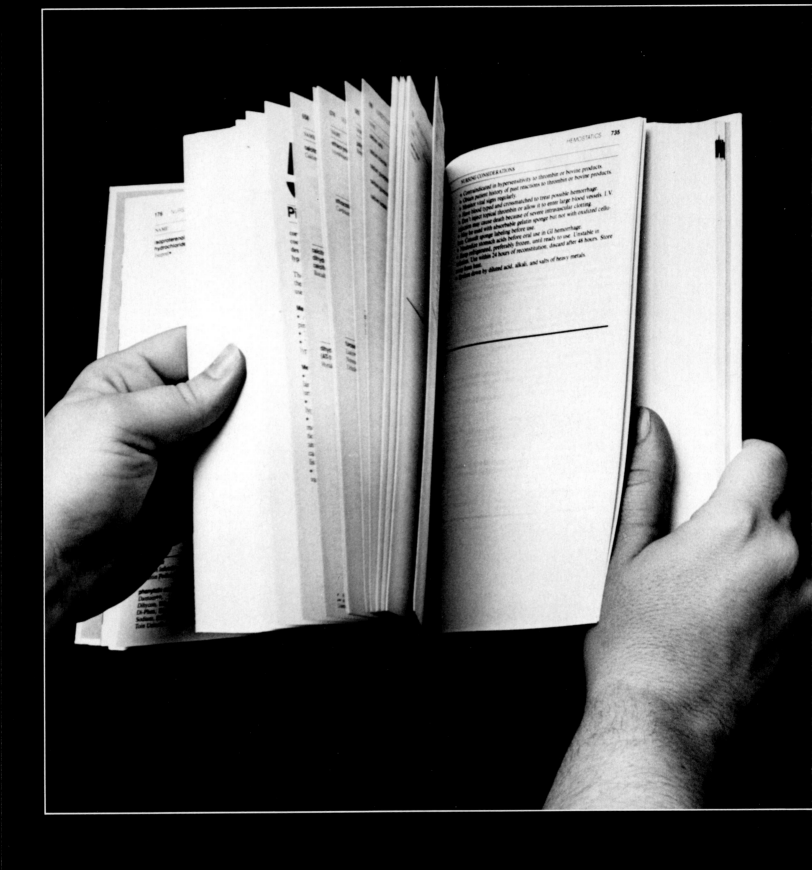

Appendices

Appendices

Nurses' guide to cardiac drugs

If your patient needs cardiac drug therapy, the doctor will order the drug, the route, and the dose. For your reference, here's a list of drugs commonly given for cardiac conditions. Refer to the *Nurse's Guide to Drugs*™ for more detailed information.

Drug	Indications	Dosage	Contraindications	Possible side effects	Special considerations
atropine sulfate	• Sinus bradycardia • Heart block	**Adults** I.V. bolus: 0.5 to 1 mg. May repeat **Children** I.V. bolus: 0.01 to 0.03 mg/kg (maximum dose)	• Tachycardia • Glaucoma • Bladder disorders	Tachycardia; flushing; dry, warm skin; increased respirations; restlessness; irritability; disorientation; incoherence; depression; urinary retention; thirst; headache; constipation	• Watch heart rate and rhythm to determine drug effects. Doctor may order an additional dose, or switch to another drug. • Watch for side effects and report signs of drug toxicity. • Store drug in a light-protected container.
bretylium tosylate Bretylol	• Life-threatening ventricular arrhythmias	**Adults and children** I.V. bolus: 5 to 10 mg/kg. Repeat every 15 to 30 minutes until a maximum dose of 30 mg/kg is delivered. *Maintenance dose* I.V. infusion: 500 mg diluted in 500 ml of 5% dextrose in water or normal saline solution, at 1 to 2 mg per minute rate. I.M.: 5 to 10 mg/kg undiluted. Repeat in 12 hours.	• Digitalis-induced arrhythmias • With caution if patient has fixed cardiac output, to avoid a severe, sudden drop in blood pressure	Hypotension (vertigo and syncope); initial transient hypertension; nausea and vomiting; transient increased heart rate; ventricular irritability	• Frequently monitor blood pressure, heart rate and rhythm. • Keep patient supine until tolerance to hypotension develops. • Potentiates some antihypotensive drugs.
diazoxide Hyperstat*	• Malignant hypertension • Impaired renal function • Hypertensive encephalopathy • Hypertension complicated by left ventricular failure • Eclampsia	**Adults** I.V. bolus: 300 mg or 5 mg/kg, administered in less than 30 seconds. May repeat at 4 to 24-hour intervals. **Children** I.V. bolus: 5 mg/kg, administered in less than 30 seconds	• Hypersensitivity to diazoxide or thiazide diuretics	Severe hyperglycemia; sodium and water retention; transient myocardial and/or cerebral ischemia; angina; transient tachycardia; palpitations; bradycardia; GI distress, including nausea, vomiting, diarrhea, abdominal discomfort, and constipation; decreased urinary output	• Have patient lie still during injection and for 30 minutes afterward. • Monitor intake and output. • Check patient's urine for sugar during therapy. • Take care to avoid extravasation. • After injection, monitor blood pressure every 5 minutes until it stabilizes, then every hour thereafter. • Make blood pressure check on ambulatory patient while he's standing.
digoxin SK-Digoxin, Lanoxin*	• Congestive heart failure • Atrial fibrillation or flutter • Termination of paroxysmal atrial tachycardia (PAT) • Supraventricular tachyarrhythmias	**Adults** *Digitalizing dose* I.V. bolus or P.O.: 0.5 to 1 mg/day in equal doses *Maintenance dose* I.V. bolus or P.O.: 0.125 to 0.5 mg/day **Children** *Less than 2 years:* *Loading dose:* P.O.: 60 to 80 mcg/kg/day in 3 divided doses *Maintenance dose:* P.O.: 20 to 25 mcg/kg/day in 2 equal doses every 12 hours	• Coronary occlusion or angina in the absence of congestive heart failure • Hypersensitivity to cardiotonic glycosides, or signs of toxicity • With caution, if the patient has ischemic heart disease; acute myocarditis; ventricular tachycardia; hypoxia or myxedemic states;	Changes in heart rate and rhythm; irritability of heart muscle and conduction system; anorexia, nausea, and vomiting; excessive salivation; abdominal pain and diarrhea; headache; fatigue; general malaise; disorientation; visual disturbances; skin reactions such as pruritis, urticaria, and facial edema	• Take apical pulses for 1 minute. Withhold drug and notify doctor if apical pulse rate is less than 60 or more than 120 in an adult, and less than 110 in a child, or according to specific order. • Monitor the digitalis-toxic patient for arrhythmias. • Monitor fluid intake and output. • Watch for signs of hypokalemia. Monitor serum potassium levels. • Observe for these position responses to drug: improved heart rate and rhythm;

*Available in both the United States and in Canada

Drug	Indications	Dosage	Contraindications	Possible side effects	Special considerations
digoxin (continued)		*Over 2 years:* *Loading dose:* 40 to 60 mcg/kg P.O. or 20 to 40 mcg/kg I.M. or I.V. Give ⅓ dose stat, then ⅓ dose every 8 hours for 2 doses *Maintenance dose:* P.O.: 10 to 15 mcg/kg divided every 12 hours I.M. or I.V.: 8 to 12 mcg/kg divided every 12 hours	Stokes-Adams syndrome; carotid sinus syndrome; emphysema; heart blocks; impaired renal or hepatic function		improved respirations; weight reduction, and diuresis.
disopyramide phosphate Norpace*	• Premature ventricular contractions • Ventricular tachycardia (not severe enough to require cardioversion)	**Adults** *Maintenance dose* P.O.: 150 to 200 mg every 6 hours *Small or thin patients, or those with renal, hepatic, or cardiac impairment:* P.O.: 100 mg every 6 hours	• Cardiogenic shock with no pacemaker • Second- or third-degree heart block • With caution if patient has congestive heart failure, urinary tract diseases, hepatic or renal impairment, myasthenia gravis, glaucoma	Decreased cardiac contractility; hypotension; increased peripheral vascular resistance; blurred vision; dry mouth; constipation; urinary retention; headache; aggravation of glaucoma.	• Check apical pulse rate before administration. Withhold drug and notify doctor if pulse rate is less than 60 beats per minute or greater than 120 beats per minute. • Instruct patient to use chewing gum and hard candy to combat dry mouth.
dopamine hydrochloride Intropin*	• Cardiogenic shock • Hypovolemic shock associated with trauma, septicemia, open heart surgery, renal failure, congestive heart failure	**Adults** I.V. infusion: 2 to 5 mcg/kg/min. Severely ill patients may receive up to 50 mcg/kg/min. **Children** I.V. infusion: 2 to 5 mcg/kg/min. May increase to no more than 20 mcg/kg/min.	• Uncorrected tachyarrhythmias • Pheochromocytoma • Ventricular fibrillation • With caution if patient has occlusive vascular disease, cold injuries, diabetic endarteritis, arterial embolism • With caution in pregnant females • With caution if patient is receiving MAO inhibitors	Cardiac arrhythmias; palpitations; widening of QRS intervals; headache; dizziness; pallor; sweating; nausea; vomiting; restlessness; tremors, weakness; respiratory difficulty; anginal-type pain; hypotension	• Keep patient under close observation, monitoring his blood pressure every 5 minutes, his cardiac conduction continuously, and his urine output hourly. Report any changes to doctor. • Check infusion site frequently for extravasation. If extravasation occurs, doctor may infiltrate site with 5 to 10 mg of phentolamine with 10 to 15 ml normal saline solution. • Use infusion pump. • Mix drug with I.V. solution just before administration. • Don't mix dopamine with other drugs.
epinephrine hydrochloride Adrenalin Chloride	• Cardiac and circulatory failure • Hypotensive states • Allergic reactions • Angioneurotic edema • Status asthmaticus	**Adults** I.M. or subcutaneously: 0.1 to 0.5 ml in 1% solution, injected slowly. May dilute to 10 ml with normal saline solution. Intracardiac: 1 ml of 1% solution. May repeat **Children** I.V. or intracardiac: 0.1 ml/kg of 1% solution, up to a maximum of 3 ml. May dilute to 10 ml with saline solution. May repeat every 5 minutes	• Shock other than anaphylactic, ventricular fibrillation, and narrow angle glaucoma • With caution in elderly patient who has angina, hypertension, or hyperthyroidism • With extreme caution if patient has degenerative heart disease	Cerebral hemorrhage; cardiac arrhythmias; palpitations; widened pulse pressure; precordial pain; headache; nervousness; vertigo, tremor; sweating, nausea; weakness; dizziness; tachycardia; hyperglycemia; EKG changes (decrease in T-wave amplitude)	• Do not expose drug to light, heat, or air. • If given intravenously, take baseline blood pressure and pulse before initiation of therapy. Then, monitor closely every minute until desired effect is reached, then every 2 minutes until patient stabilizes. After patient stabilizes, monitor blood pressure every 15 minutes. • If patient experiences sharp increase in blood pressure, administer rapid-acting vasodilators, as ordered.

*Available in both the United States and in Canada

Appendices

Nurses' guide to cardiac drugs   continued

Drug	Indications	Dosage	Contraindications	Possible side effects	Special considerations
ethacrynate sodium Edecrin*	• Congestive heart failure • Pulmonary edema • Edema associated with nephrotic syndrome • Hepatic cirrhosis • Ascites • Idiopathic edema and lymphedema • Patient resistant to less potent diuretics	**Adults** I.V. bolus: 50 to 100 mg given slowly. May be repeated at another site P.O.: 50 to 200 mg daily **Children** I.V. bolus: 1 mg/kg per dose P.O.: 25 mg daily. Can be increased in 25 mg increments.	• Anuria. Severe renal damage • Infants • With caution if patient has diabetes, hepatic cirrhosis, history of gout	Hypokalemia; hyponatremia; reduced blood volume; deafness; tetany; hypochloremic alkalosis; malaise; GI distress; GI bleeding, especially with concomitant heparin therapy; hyperuricemia; hyperglycemia, glycosuria; blurred vision, confusion; fever, chills, weakness, fatigue; postural hypotension; muscle cramps	• Monitor patient's intake and output levels and his serum electrolyte levels. Weigh him daily. • Watch for signs of hypokalemia. • Watch for signs of excessive diuresis, especially in elderly patient. • Give oral dose in a.m. to prevent nocturia.
furosemide Lasix*	• Edema, associated with congestive heart failure • Nephrotic syndrome • Hepatic cirrhosis • Ascites • Hypertension • Acute pulmonary edema • Severe hypercalcemia	**Adults** *Edema* P.O.: 20 to 80 mg daily. May increase by 40 mg every 8 hours until diuretic effect attained I.V. bolus: 20 to 40 mg over 1 to 2 minutes. Increase by 20 mg every 2 hours. *Hypertensive crisis* I.V. bolus: 100 to 200 mg over 2 minutes. *Hypercalcemia* I.V. bolus: 80 to 100 mg every hour until serum calcium levels are normal. Then, 120 mg P.O. **Children** P.O.: 2 mg/kg/day, as ordered. Increase dose by 1 to 2 mg/kg in 6 to 8 hours. Maximum dose 6 mg/kg daily	• Anuria • Hypersensitivity to drug • Severe renal disease associated with azotemia and oliguria • Hepatic coma, associated with electrolyte depletion • Pregnancy	Electrolyte imbalance, hyperkalemia, dehydration; metabolic alkalosis; blurred vision; postural hypotension; nausea, vomiting, diarrhea; weakness, fatigue, dizziness; muscle cramps, bladder spasms; tinnitus; urinary frequency and bladder spasms; dermatitis	• Monitor blood pressure closely. • Monitor patient's serum electrolyte levels as well as blood sugar and uric acid levels. • May cause an allergic reaction in the sulfonamide-sensitive patient. • With elderly patient, stay alert for signs of excessive diuresis, vascular thrombosis and embolism.
hydralazine hydrochloride Apresoline*	• Essential hypertensive states, including those associated with pregnancy • Early malignant hypertension	**Adults** I.V. bolus or I.M.: 20 to 40 mg, administered slowly and repeated if necessary every 6 hours P.O.: 10 mg four times a day, gradually increased to 50 mg daily **Children** I.V. or I.M.: 1.7 to 3.5 mg/kg/day. P.O.: 0.75 mg/kg in 4 divided doses.	• Essential hypertension • Severe congestive heart failure	Orthostatic hypotension; tachycardia; headache, dizziness; angina; GI disturbances, including nausea, vomiting, and diarrhea; decreased urine volume; thrombocytopenia, leukopenic eosinophilia; peripheral neuritis; rash; sodium retention	• Monitor blood pressure and heart rate closely. • Watch for postural hypotension. • Instruct patient to avoid making sudden change in position that could cause dizziness and possible injury. • If given orally, advise patient to take drug with meals. • Tell outpatient to avoid drinking alcohol while on medication.

*Available in both the United States and in Canada

Drug	Indications	Dosage	Contraindications	Possible side effects	Special considerations
isoproterenol hydrochloride Isuprel*	• Cardiac standstill • Adams-Stokes and carotid sinus syndromes • Bradycardia • AV heart block	**Adults** I.V. infusion: 2 mg in 500 ml of 5% dextrose in water. Adjust infusion according to heart rate I.V. bolus: .02 to .06 mg, then .01 to .2 mg as necessary I.M.: 0.2 mg initially, then 0.2 to 1 mg as necessary Intracardiac: 0.02 mg (in extreme cases) **Children** I.V. infusion: 1 mg in 100 ml of 5% dextrose in water. Give at 0.1 to 0.5 mcg/kg/min. Adjust rate to patient's response.	• Tachycardia caused by digitalis intoxication • Preexisting arrhythmias • With caution if patient has coronary insufficiency, diabetes, hyperthyroidism	Tachycardia; palpitations; bronchial edema; flushing; headache; cardiac arrhythmias; chest pain; tremors; anxiety; fatigue; nausea and vomiting; swelling of parotid glands with prolonged use	• Closely monitor patient's heart rate and rhythm, blood pressure, CVP, EKG, arterial blood gases, and urinary output. If heart rate exceeds 110 beats per minute (bpm), slow down or discontinue infusion. A heart rate over 130 bpm may trigger ventricular arrhythmias. • When administering by I.V. infusion, use an infusion pump.
lidocaine hydrochloride Xylocaine*	• Ventricular tachycardia • Acute ventricular arrhythmias secondary to myocardial infarction or cardiotonic glycosides	**Adults** I.V. bolus: 50 to 100 mg at 25 to 50 mg/min. May repeat in 3 to 5 minutes. Maximum dose per hour, 200 to 300 mg I.V. infusion: 1 to 2 gm in 500 ml 5% dextrose in water at 1 to 4 mg per minute. I.M.: 200 to 300 mg, in deltoid muscle only **Children** I.V. bolus: 1 mg/kg. May repeat, but not to exceed 3 mg/kg daily. I.V. infusion: 1 gm in 1,000 ml 5% dextrose in water, at 20 to 40 mcg/kg/min.	• Hypersensitivity to amide-type local anesthetics • Adams-Stokes syndrome • Complete or second-degree heart block • With caution if the patient has liver or severe kidney disease; congestive heart failure; marked hypoxia; severe respiratory depression; shock	Dizziness, restlessness, apprehension tinnitus, visual disturbances, hearing loss; vomiting; difficulty breathing or swallowing; twitching, tremors, convulsions; hypotension; cardiovascular collapse; cardiac conduction disorders; bradycardia; cardiac and respiratory arrest; numbness in extremities, lips, or tongue	• Monitor patient's heartbeat and blood pressure during administration. • Watch for side effects and report any reaction to doctor. • When administering by I.V. infusion, use an infusion pump. • For antiarrhythmic therapy, don't use lidocaine with epinephrine added. • If toxic signs, such as dizziness, appear, stop administration at once. Continued infusion could lead to convulsions and coma.
mannitol Osmitrol*	• Oliguria or acute renal failure • Elevated intraocular pressure or intracranial pressure • Also, to test renal function and induce diuresis after drug overdose	**Adults and children over age 12** *Oliguria* I.V. bolus: 12.5 gm as a 15% or 20% solution over 5 minutes I.V. infusion: 50 to 100 gm as a 5% to 25% solution. Maximum dose is 100 gm/day for patient excreting less than 100 ml/hr *Edema* I.V. infusion: 100 gm in a 20% solution over 2 to 6 hours	• Anuria • Impaired renal function or cardiac function • Pulmonary congestion • Severe congestive heart failure (CHF) • Severe dehydration • Active intracranial bleeding	Nasal congestion; thirst; mild anginalike chest pain; localized edema at injection site; dehydration; blurred vision; urinary retention; uricosuria; urticaria; hyponatremia; hypokalemia; hyperkalemia; acidosis; rebound increase in intracranial pressure	• Response considered adequate if urine output's 30 to 50 ml/hr. • Monitor hourly fluid intake and output, and blood pressure, pulse, and central venous pressure (CVP). • Weigh daily. • Observe patient for signs of water intoxication and electrolyte imbalance. • If mannitol solution has crystalized, redissolve it in a hot water bath. • When administering I.V., always use an in-line filter.

*Available in both the United States and in Canada

Appendices

Nurses' guide to cardiac drugs continued

Drug	Indications	Dosage	Contraindications	Possible side effects	Special considerations
metaraminol bitartrate Aramine*	• To prevent and treat hypotension due to shock	**Adults** I.M. or subcutaneously: 2 to 10 mg I.V. bolus: 0.5 to 5 mg followed by I.V. infusion I.V. infusion: 15 to 100 mg in 500 ml 5% dextrose in water or normal saline solution, administered at rate sufficient to maintain blood pressure at desired level. **Children** I.V. bolus: 0.01 mg/kg I.V. infusion: 1 mg in 25 ml 5% dextrose in water. Administer at rate sufficient to maintain adequate blood pressure. I.M.: 0.1 mg/kg, as necessary.	• Pulmonary edema; cardiac arrest; during anesthesia with cyclopropane and halogenated hydrocarbons; peripheral or mesenteric thrombosis • With caution in patients with heart disease, hypertension, thyroid disease, diabetes, cirrhosis, malaria, or with patients receiving digitalis	Cerebral hemorrhage; cardiac arrhythmias; precordial pain; headache, vertigo, tremor; hypertension; hypotension, nervousness; sweating, nausea; pallor, and respiratory difficulty; hyperglycemia; decreased urinary output	• Observe for side effects and notify doctor. • Obtain baseline blood pressure reading. Then, monitor every 15 minutes during administration. • Closely monitor diabetic patient. Drug may cause hyperglycemia. Adjust insulin dosages as necessary. • When administering by I.V. infusion, use an infusion pump. Try to avoid extravasation. If it occurs, stop infusion, and call doctor. • When discontinuing therapy, gradually slow infusion rate. • Do not mix with other drugs. • Keep atropine on hand to treat reflux bradycardia, phentolamine to decrease vasopressor effects, and propranolol to treat arrhythmias.
methyldopa Aldomet*	• Mild to severe hypertension	**Adults** *Initial dose* P.O.: 250 mg every 2 to 4 hours for first 24 hours. Then increase as necessary every 2 days. *Maintenance dose* P.O.: 500 mg to 2 gm daily in 2 to 4 divided doses with a maximum dose of 3 gm/day I.V. infusion: 250 to 500 mg in 5% dextrose in water, given over 30 to 60 minutes **Children** P.O.: 10 mg/kg in 2 to 3 divided doses, with maximum dose of 65 mg/kg/day.	• Drug sensitivity • Labile and mild hypertension • Active hepatic disease • Pheochromocytoma • With caution if patient is receiving other antihypertensive drugs or MAO inhibitors.	Drowsiness, vertigo, headache, syncope, weakness; orthostatic hypertension; aggravation of angina; sodium retention; edema; anemia; fever; jaundice; bradycardia; nasal stuffiness; dry mouth; GI distress, black tongue; impotence; rash; arthralgia, myalgia, paresthesia, parkinsonism	• Monitor blood pressure closely, especially before administering another dose. • Monitor fluid intake and output. Notify doctor if patient has reduced urine output. • Weigh patient daily. • Instruct patient to avoid sudden position changes, to prevent orthostatic hypertension. • Tell patient to avoid alcohol. Encourage him to follow prescribed diet.
nitroglycerin Nitrostat*, Nitrol ointment	• Acute angina attacks • Coronary insufficiency • Hypertension • Paroxysmal nocturnal dyspnea • Prophylaxis against chronic anginal attacks	**Adults** Sublingually: 0.15 to 0.6 mg (gr.1/400 to gr. 1/100) every 5 minutes until pain is relieved. For chronic anginal attacks, one sustained-release capsule every 8 to 12 hours Topically: ½″ of 2% ointment, increase in ½″ increments until headache occurs. Usual dose 1 to 2 inches.	• Sensitivity to nitrates • Head trauma, cerebral hemorrhage • Myocardial infarction • Severe anemia • With caution if patient has glaucoma or is hypotensive	Headache; orthostatic hypotension; nausea, vomiting, dizziness, weakness; syncope; drug rash; palpitations; tachycardia; sublingual burning	• Administer with patient in sitting or lying position, to prevent postural hypotension. • Get new supply of drug every 3 months. • Remove cotton from container, since it absorbs drug. • Patient may take aspirin or acetaminophen for headaches. • Instruct patient to store drug in dark, cool place. • Instruct patient to avoid taking drug with alcohol.

*Available in both the United States and in Canada

Drug	Indications	Dosage	Contraindications	Possible side effects	Special considerations
nitroglycerin (continued)					• To apply ointment, spread in uniform, thin layer on a nonhairy area. Cover with plastic wrap to enhance absorption.
nitroprusside sodium Nipride*	• Hypertensive emergencies • Cardiac pump failure	**Adults** I.V. infusion: 50 mg in 500 to 1,000 ml 5% dextrose in water delivered at 0.5 to 10 mcg/kg/min. Average dose 3 mcg/kg/min **Children** I.V. infusion: 0.3 to 5.7 mcg/kg/min, as ordered.	• Compensatory hypertension	Transitory CNS symptoms, such as restlessness, agitation, absent reflexes, and muscle twitching; cyanide toxicity; vomiting, nausea; skin rash; excessive hypotensive effects	• Due to light sensitivity, wrap I.V. container in opaque material, such as aluminum foil. • Label wrapped container with mixture, time hung, and time to be replaced. • Reconstitute with 5% dextrose in water only. Never mix any other drug with Nipride solution. • Discard and replace solution every 4 hours, or if it turns any color other than brown. • Administer with infusion pump. • Monitor blood pressure every 5 minutes. Stop Nipride if severe hypotension occurs. • Tissue irritation can occur with extravasation. • May cause cyanide toxicity (thiocyanate). Blood levels should be checked every 72 hours.
norepinephrine, formerly called **levarterenol bitartrate** Levophed*	• To treat acute hypotensive states caused by trauma, central vasomotor depression, or myocardial infarction	**Adults** I.V. infusion: Initially 8 to 12 mcg/min. Then adjust to maintain blood pressure at desired level. Average maintenance dose 2 to 4 mcg/min.	• Peripheral vascular thrombosis • Hypoxia • Pregnancy • Hypotension from blood volume deficiency • With caution if patient has heart disease or obstruction of urinary tract, hypertension, or hyperthyroidism • Do not administer with cyclopropane and halothane anesthesia (can cause fatal arrhythmias) • With caution if patient is receiving MAO inhibitors or tricyclic antidepressants	Cerebral hemorrhage; cardiac arrhythmias such as bradycardia, or ventricular tachycardia; precordial pain; excess CNS stimulation, headache, nervousness, tremors, insomnia; sweating; nausea; pallor; respiratory difficulties	• Take a baseline blood pressure reading before administration. • Check blood pressure every 2 minutes during administration until desired level is obtained. • Take blood pressure frequently after administration to assure that desired drug level is maintained. • Administer via large vein, using infusion pump. Try to avoid extravasation. If it occurs, stop infusion, and infiltrate area with 5 to 10 mg phentolamine and 10 to 15 ml normal saline solution. • When discontinuing therapy, slow infusion rate gradually. Monitor vital signs. • Administer in dextrose and saline solution; saline solution alone is not recommended. • Incompatible with whole blood and plasma. Administer separately. • Use atropine to treat reflex bradycardia and propranolol to treat arrhythmias.

*Available in both the United States and in Canada

Appendices

Nurses' guide to cardiac drugs   continued

Drug	Indications	Dosage	Contraindications	Possible side effects	Special considerations
phenytoin sodium Dilantin*	• Cardiac arrhythmias (especially those induced by digitalis) • Ventricular arrhythmias unresponsive to lidocaine or procainamide • Arrhythmias induced by cardiac glycosides	**Adults** P.O.: 1 gm in divided doses over 24 hours. Then, 500 mg daily for 48 hours. Then, 300 mg daily thereafter. I.V. bolus: 250 mg given slowly over 5 minutes. Do not exceed rate of 50 mg/min. **Children** P.O. or I.V. bolus: 3 to 8 mg/kg	• Cardiac disturbances, for example, heart block, sinus bradycardia or Stokes-Adams syndrome • Lactating females • Hypersensitivity to drug • With caution if patient has history of asthma or other allergies, impaired renal function, congestive heart failure • With caution if patient is receiving oral anticoagulants	Ataxia; uncoordinated movements; dizziness; headache; increased motor activity; hallucinations; fatigue, insomnia; apathy; hypoglycemia; visual disturbances; tinnitus; serious cardiovascular effects, including hypotension, shock, cardiovascular collapse, heart block; GI disturbances; gingival hyperplasia; blood disturbances	• Do not mix drug with 5% dextrose in water, or drug will precipitate. • Drug may color urine pink, red, or reddish-brown. • Monitor blood pressure and EKG closely. • Give drug with food to minimize gastric irritation. • Serum levels over 20 mcg/ml may be toxic. • Warn patients not to drink alcohol when taking this drug.
procainamide hydrochloride Pronestyl*	• Premature ventricular contractions • Ventricular tachycardia • Atrial arrhythmias unresponsive to quinidine • Paroxysmal atrial tachycardia (PAT)	**Adults** *Ventricular tachycardia, PAT, atrial arrhythmias* I.V. bolus: 100 mg every 5 minutes no faster than 25 to 50 mg/min until arrhythmia disappears or until 1 gm has been given. When arrhythmias disappear, give I.V. infusion of 2 to 6 mg/min. I.M.: 0.5 to 1 gm every 4 to 8 hours until oral therapy begins. *Atrial fibrillation and PAT Initial dose* P.O.: 1 to 1.25 gm *Maintenance dose* P.O.: 0.5 to 1 gm every 4 to 6 hours *Ventricular tachycardia Initial dose:* P.O.: 1 gm *Maintenance dose:* P.O.: 250 to 500 mg every 3 hours	• Sensitivity to procainamide or procaine • Complete heart block, second- or third-degree heart block unassisted by pacemaker • Blood dyscrasias • Myasthenia gravis • With caution if patient has bronchial asthma; congestive heart failure; conduction disturbances; cardiotonic glycosides intoxication; hepatic or renal insufficiency	Hypotension, especially when drug is given I.V.; cardiac disturbances, including bradycardia, partial or complete heart block, asystole, extrasystole, ventricular fibrillation with parenteral administration, circulatory collapse; drug induced lupus; urticaria; fever, chills; weakness, depression; psychosis; hallucinations; confusion, convulsions; depression; allergic reactions; GI disturbances, including anorexia; bitter taste, nausea, vomiting, and diarrhea	• Keep patient supine during I.V. infusion. • Administer drug using I.V. infusion pump. • Monitor blood pressure constantly. Report drop of 15 mm Hg or more in blood pressure during administration. • Have on hand drug such as Levophed* to counteract hypotensive effect. • Observe monitor for prolonged Q-T and Q-R intervals, heart block, or increased arrhythmias. If these occur, discontinue infusion, obtain rhythm strip, and notify doctor immediately.
propranolol hydrochloride Inderal*	• Supraventricular, atrial, and ventricular arrhythmias • Hypertension • Angina	**Adults** *Initial dose* I.V. bolus: 1 to 3 mg diluted in 50 ml 5% dextrose in water or normal saline solution, at rate not to exceed 1 mg/min. Dose may be repeated in 2 minutes, then every 4 hours.	• Diabetes • Sinus bradycardia • Heart block greater than first degree • Cardiogenic shock • Right ventricular failure	CHF or circulatory collapse; hypotension; cardiac disturbances, including bradycardia, angina, asystole, AV heart block; GI disturbances; CNS disturbances,	• Take apical pulse rate before administration. If pulse is below 50 bpm, withhold drug and notify doctor. • Auscultate patient's lungs for rales and his heart for gallop rhythm during administration. If found, notify doctor. • Have atropine on hand to

*Available in both the United States and in Canada

Drug	Indications	Dosage	Contraindications	Possible side effects	Special considerations
propranolol hydrochloride (continued)		*Maintenance dose* P.O.: 10 to 80 mg every 2 to 4 hours, with maximum dose of 320 mg/day	• Bronchial asthma • With caution if patient has renal or hepatic dysfunction; left ventricular heart failure; acute myocardial infarction; arrhythmias induced by digitalis toxicity; respiratory disease • With caution after cardioversion	including hallucinations, uncoordinated movements, vertigo, syncope, dizziness, insomnia, confusion, and depression; rashes; urinary retention; peripheral vascular insufficiency; bronchospasms, wheezing; blood sugar abnormalities	counteract possible bradycardia • Observe diabetic patient for insulin shock (propranolol masks characteristic signs of hypoglycemia, including tachycardia and sweating). • When stopping therapy, slow infusion rate gradually.
quinidine sulfate Extentabs*	• Atrial flutter or fibrillation • Atrial and ventricular arrhythmias • Ventricular ectopia • Congestive heart failure (CHF) • Paroxysmal supraventricular tachycardia • Maintenance after cardioversion	**Adults** *Atrial flutter and fibrillation* P.O.: 200 mg every 2 to 3 hours for 5 to 8 doses; maximum 3 to 4 gm daily. *Paroxysmal supraventricular tachycardia* I.M.: 400 to 600 mg every 2 to 3 hours until toxic signs develop *Congestive heart failure* P.O.: 200 mg every 6 hours *All other arrhythmias* P.O.: 50 to 200 mg. Then, 200 to 400 mg every 4 to 6 hours **Children** P.O.: 2 mg/kg, then 3 to 6 mg/kg every 2 to 3 hours for 5 doses.	• Cardiotonic glycosides toxicity when AV conduction's impaired • AV block with AV nodal or idioventricular pacemaker • With caution if the patient has myasthenia gravis; muscular weakness; respiratory distress; bronchial asthma	Bradycardia; CHF; angina; partial or total heart block; EKG changes such as widening of QRS complex, notched P waves, widened Q-T interval, or S-T segment depression; severe hypotension; asystole; circulatory collapse; ventricular tachycardia; cinchonism; dyspnea, respiratory paralysis; cyanosis, syncope; urticaria; blood disorders; GI disturbances; CNS disturbances, such as confusion, vertigo, apprehension, convulsions, headache, tremors, cold sweats, salivation, flushing, visual disturbances	• Take apical pulse rate and blood pressure before administration. • Administer drug with meals or antacids to reduce GI side effects. Amphojel* is the antacid of choice because it doesn't affect quinidine absorption. • Do not use discolored liquid. • Have lidocaine on hand to treat quinidine-induced arrhythmias.
sodium bicarbonate	• Cardiac arrest • Metabolic acidosis	**Adults** *Cardiac arrest* I.V. bolus: 1 to 3 mEq/kg, initially; may repeat in 10 minutes. Further dose based on arterial blood gas (ABG) measurement. *Metabolic acidosis* I.V. infusion: 2 to 5 mEq over a 4 to 8 hour period. **Children** *Cardiac arrest* I.V. bolus: 1 mEq/kg. Further dose based on ABG measurement. Not to exceed 8 mEq/kg/day	• No contraindications for life-threatening emergencies • Contraindicated in patients with hypertension, renal disease, tendency toward edema, in those losing chlorides by vomiting or from continuous GI suction, in those receiving diuretics known to produce hypochloremic alkalosis, and in those on salt restriction.	GI disturbances, such as increased stomach acid secretion, gastric distention, abdominal cramps, anorexia, nausea, and vomiting; dizziness, convulsions; thirst; diminished respirations; renal calculi or crystals; with overdose, alkalosis, hypernatremia, hyperosmolarity	• May be added to I.V. solution, unless solution contains epinephrine or norepinephrine. • Do not infuse through I.V. line containing calcium, or the drug will precipitate. • Obtain arterial blood gas (ABG) and serum electrolytes measurements during administration and report changes.

*Available in both the United States and in Canada

Appendices

Nurses' guide to EKG interpretations

On page 47 you learned how to read an EKG. Diagnosing your patient's condition using the EKG is the doctor's job. But you should be familiar enough with EKG waveforms to know when your patient requires immediate attention. That's why we've included this chart. It features all the basic EKG readings you're likely to encounter, as well as the probable interpretation.

HEART RHYTHM		HEART RATE		ELECTRICAL CONDUCTION	CONFIGURATION	INTERPRETATION
Atrial	Ventricular	Atrial	Ventricular			
Regular	Regular	60 to 100 beats per minute	60 to 100 beats per minute	P-R intervals normal; P wave for every QRS complex	P wave normal; QRS complex normal	Normal sinus rhythm
Regular	Regular	60 beats per minute or less	60 beats per minute or less	P-R intervals normal; P wave for every QRS complex	P wave normal; QRS complex normal	Sinus bradycardia
Regular	Regular	100 to 150 beats per minute	100 to 150 beats per minute	P-R intervals normal; P wave for every QRS complex	P wave normal; QRS complex normal	Sinus tachycardia
Irregular	Irregular	60 to 100 beats per minute	60 to 100 beats per minute	P-R intervals normal; P wave for every QRS complex	P wave normal; QRS complex normal	Sinus arrhythmia
Regular or irregular	Regular or irregular	60 to 100 beats per minute	60 to 100 beats per minute	P-R intervals may vary, but no more than 0.2 seconds; P wave for every QRS complex	P wave variable; QRS complex normal	Wandering pacemaker
Irregular (due to decreased PQRS complex)	Irregular (due to decreased PQRS complex)	Variable	Variable	P-R intervals normal	P wave normal; QRS complex normal	Sinus pause
Irregular (due to premature P waves)	Irregular (due to premature P waves)	Variable	Variable	P-R intervals extended because of premature P waves; P wave for every QRS complex	Premature P waves may be inverted or irregularly shaped	Premature atrial contractions (PAC)
Irregular (due to premature P waves)	Irregular (due to premature P waves)	Variable	Variable	P-R intervals normal when they can be measured; Premature P waves not followed by QRS complex	Premature P waves may be inverted, irregularly shaped, or hidden in QRS complex or T wave ; QRS complex normal	Nonconducted premature atrial contraction
Regular	Regular	150 to 250 beats per minute	150 to 250 beats per minute	P-R intervals normal or prolonged; P wave usually followed by QRS complex	P wave abnormal or inverted but shape stays constant; P wave sometimes merges with T wave; QRS complex normal	Paroxysmal atrial tachycardia (PAT)
Regular	Regular or irregular	250 to 300 beats per minute	Variable	P-R waves constant or variable; QRS complex follows flutter wave, but not all flutter waves are followed by QRS complex	Saw-toothed P waves; QRS complex normal	Atrial flutter
Irregular	Irregular	Over 400 beats per minute	Under 100 beats per minute: controlled Over 100 beats per minute: uncontrolled	P-R intervals can't be measured; P waves indistinct	P wave appears as wavy baseline; QRS complex normal	Atrial fibrillation
Regular (if P wave is visible)	Regular (if P wave is visible)	40 to 60 beats per minute	40 to 60 beats per minute	P-R intervals shorter than normal, when they can be measured; P wave may precede, follow, or be hidden in QRS complex	P wave usually inverted; QRS complex normal	Junctional rhythm

HEART RHYTHM		HEART RATE		ELECTRICAL CONDUCTION	CONFIGURATION	INTERPRETATION
Atrial	Ventricular	Atrial	Ventricular			
Regular or irregular	Regular or irregular	Variable	Variable	Premature P wave shortens P-R intervals; Premature P wave may precede, follow, or be hidden in the QRS complex	Premature P wave otherwise normal; may be inverted or hidden; QRS complex normal	Premature junctional contractions
Regular (if P wave is visible)	Regular	Over 60 beats per minute (if P wave is visible)	Over 60 beats per minute	P-R intervals shorter than normal, if measurable; P wave may precede, follow, or be hidden in the QRS complex	P wave different than sinus P wave, if visible; QRS complex normal	Junctional tachycardia
Regular (if visible)	Regular or irregular	Variable	20 to 40 beats per minute	P-R intervals variable; P wave relationship to QRS complex variable	P wave normal when visible; QRS complex abnormal and widened; T wave usually in opposite direction of QRS complex	Ventricular rhythm
Regular or irregular	Irregular	Variable	Variable	P-R intervals shorter than normal, when they can be measured; P wave relationship to QRS complex variable	P wave constant or variable; QRS complex abnormal and widened; T wave usually in opposite direction of QRS complex	Premature ventricular contraction
Regular (if visible)	Regular	Variable	40 to 100 beats per minute	P-R intervals variable; P wave relationship to QRS complex variable	P wave normal when visible; QRS complex wide and bizarre; T wave opposite of QRS complex	Accelerated ventricular rhythm
Regular	Regular or irregular	Variable	100 to 270 beats per minute	P-R intervals variable; P wave relationship to QRS complex variable	P wave normal when visible; QRS wider than normal, may vary; T wave opposite of QRS complex	Ventricular tachycardia
Not visible	Irregular	Not determinable	Extremely rapid	P-R intervals can't be determined; P wave relationship to QRS complex not visible	P wave not visible; No defined QRS complex	Ventricular fibrillation
Regular (if present)	Not present	Variable	None present	Nonexistent; P wave relationship to QRS complex not visible	P wave normal (if visible); QRS complex not visible	Ventricular standstill
Regular	Regular	Variable with underlying rhythm	Same as atrial	P-R intervals over 0.2 seconds; P wave for every QRS complex	P wave normal; QRS complex normal	First-degree AV block
Regular	Irregular	Variable, but greater than ventricular	Variable	P-R intervals progressively prolonged; P wave before every QRS complex, but QRS complex may not follow every P wave	P wave normal; QRS complex normal	Second-degree AV block (Wenckebach)
Regular	Regular, except for pause caused by missing QRS complex	Variable, but greater than ventricular	Variable	P-R intervals normal or prolonged, but consistent; P wave before every QRS complex, but QRS complex may not follow every P wave	P wave normal; QRS complex normal or 0.12 seconds greater than normal	Second-degree AV block (Mobitz II)
Regular	Regular	Twice that of ventricular	Variable	P-R intervals normal or prolonged, but constant; two P waves for every QRS complex	P wave normal; QRS complex normal	Second-degree AV block (2:1 conduction)
Regular	Regular	Variable, but greater than ventricular	Variable	P-R intervals variable with no pattern; no relationship between P wave and QRS complex	P wave normal; QRS complex normal or abnormal	Third-degree AV block

Appendices

Nurses' guide to diagnostic blood work

Your patient has a cardiac condition. How can diagnostic blood work help his doctor treat him effectively? That depends on the test. The doctor may order tests to determine levels of cholesterol, triglyceride and high-density lipoprotein (HDL) in the patient's bloodstream. Getting this information helps him assess the patient's risk factors. Or, if the doctor suspects that the patient's suffered a myocardial infarction (MI), the doctor may order serial studies of specific enzymes to confirm the diagnosis. To diagnose an MI with even greater accuracy, he may order cardiac isoenzyme studies. On these pages, you'll learn the basics of what these tests can tell you.

Cardiac enzymes and isoenzymes: Critical clues

Enzymes are catalytic proteins that vary in function and concentration, depending on the tissue in which they appear. Since damaged tissue (including the myocardium) releases enzymes into the blood, enzyme studies may tell you what organ's damaged, and to what extent.

Take a look at the chart below. It describes three enzymes helpful in diagnosing heart tissue damage. As you see, however, these enzymes appear in other tissues besides the myocardium. To make sure an elevated enzyme level indicates myocardial damage (and not damage to some other tissue), the doctor may order cardiac isoenzyme studies.

Both of the enzymes lactic dehydrogenase (LDH) and creatine phosphokinase (CPK) may be divided into isoenzymes, or distinct subgroups. (No isoenzymes are known for SGOT.) Five isoenzymes are known for LDH (LDH_1 through LDH_5); three isoenzymes are known for CPK (CPK_1, CPK_2, and CPK_3). By determining which isoenzyme levels are elevated, the doctor may be able to pinpoint damaged tissue.

Let's consider LDH isoenzymes first. Elevation of one or more LDH isoenzymes suggests a specific disorder. Elevation of LDH_1 and LDH_2 indicates myocardial infarction; elevation of LDH_3 indicates pulmonary infarction; and elevation of LDH_4 and LDH_5 indicates liver disease.

Note: Some laboratories routinely check hydroxybutyrate dehydrogenase (HBD) levels as an indirect measure of LDH_1 and LDH_2. The chart on the opposite page shows the close correlation of HBD with LDH_1 and LDH_2.

Here are approximate normal percentages for LDH isoenzymes:
- LDH_1 - 20%
- LDH_2 - 35%
- LDH_3 - 20%
- LDH_4 - 15%
- LDH_5 - 10%

CPK isoenzymes are also highly reliable in identifying heart tissue damage. CPK isoenzymes found in the blood are identified as follows:
- CPK_1, or BB (originates in brain)
- CPK_2, or MB (originates in heart muscle)
- CPK_3, or MM (originates in skeletal muscle).

Normally, only CPK_3 is present in blood. So, CPK_2, when it appears, strongly suggests heart muscle damage. (Likewise, the appearance of CPK_1 suggests brain damage or disease.) As a general rule, CPK_2 is

Learning cardiac enzyme basics

Cardiac enzyme	Tissues containing this enzyme	Cardiac conditions causing enzyme elevation in blood	Other conditions causing enzyme elevation in blood	Drugs causing enzyme elevation in blood
SGOT (serum glutamic-oxalo-acetic transaminase) Normal values: 0 to 36 IU/liter (international units per liter)	Heart muscle, liver, skeletal muscle, kidney, brain, pancreas, spleen, lungs, red blood cells	Myocardial infarction, severe arrhythmias, severe angina, cardiac catheterization	Liver disease, acute pancreatitis, severe skeletal muscle trauma, severe burns, acute renal disease, acute hemolytic anemia, brain trauma, muscular dystrophy	Aspirin, codeine, cortisone, cholinergics, theophylline, vitamin A, meperidine, hydralazine, erythromycin, morphine, tolbutamide, griseofulvin
LDH (lactic dehydrogenase) Normal values: 120 to 340 IU/liter	Widely distributed in body tissue, including heart muscle, liver, kidney, brain, skeletal muscle, lungs, and erythrocytes	Myocardial infarction	Pulmonary infarction, megaloblastic anemia, cancer, shock, anoxia, hemolytic anemia, infectious mononucleosis, muscular dystrophy	Codeine, clofibrate, meperidine, mithramycin, morphine, procainamide
CPK (creatine phosphokinase) Normal values: Male: 20 to 140 IU/liter; Female: 10 to 100 IU/liter	Heart muscle, skeletal muscle, brain	Myocardial infarction, cardiac surgery, cardiac defibrillation	Muscular dystrophy, dermatomyositis, myxedema, delirium tremens, hypokalemia, CNS trauma, pulmonary infarction, acute psychosis. *Important:* If the patient's received any intramuscular injections within the past week, make sure you note this on the laboratory request form. Muscular damage during injection may cause false elevation of test results.	Amphotericin B, clofibrate, and salicylates (given in high dosages)

Acknowledgements

detectable in the bloodstream several hours after an MI, and remains detectable for several days.

Testing for risk factors

How can diagnostic blood work help you assess the patient's risk factors? By determining his fasting blood-fat (lipid) levels. As you know, high levels of two blood fats—cholesterol and triglyceride—may contribute significantly to coronary artery disease. If your patient's cholesterol and/or triglyceride levels are above normal, he'll need to modify his diet and reduce other risk factors.

What serum cholesterol and triglyceride levels indicate that your patient's at risk? Consider these figures as danger signs:
• a serum cholesterol level above 250 mg/100 ml (normal: 150 to 250 mg/100 ml)
• a serum triglyceride level above 150 mg/100 ml (normal: 40 to 150 mg/100 ml).

Note: These drugs may elevate cholesterol levels: ACTH, aminopyrine, androgens, bile salts, bromides, clofibrate, cortisone, and epinephrine.

A new lab test helps the doctor assess risk factors by comparing cholesterol levels to high-density lipoprotein (HDL) levels. HDL seems to *reduce* the risk of coronary artery disease by inhibiting the absorption of cholesterol by arterial wall cells. In addition, HDL increases the rate at which cholesterol leaves these cells.

What's a desirable ratio? A ratio of 3.5 (or fewer) units of cholesterol to 1 unit of HDL is considered low risk. A ratio of 5 units of cholesterol to 1 unit of HDL represents a standard risk. As the ratio of cholesterol to HDL rises above 5 to 1, your patient's risk increases.

Since exercise seems to raise HDL levels, active people often have favorable cholesterol-to-HDL ratios. That's one reason why the doctor will want your patient to continue an exercise program after discharge, and to maintain a low-cholesterol diet.

Note: Women generally have higher HDL levels than men. This may be one reason they're less likely to develop coronary artery disease.

We'd like to thank the following people and companies for their help with this PHOTOBOOK.

BURDICK CORPORATION
Hackensack, N.J.
Jules Pitsker,
District Manager

CORATOMIC, INC.
Indiana, Pa.
John T. Hagy, President

DATASCOPE CORPORATION
Paramus, N.J.

HEALTHCO, INC.
Reading, Pa.
Al Szymborski, CMR

HEWLETT-PACKARD CO.
Waltham, Mass.

THE JOBST INSTITUTE, INC.
Toledo, Ohio

KONTRON CARDIOVASCULAR, INC.
Formerly *Avco Medical Products*
Everett, Mass.

MEDTRONIC, INC.
Minneapolis, Minn.

NARCO AIR-SHIELDS
Division of NARCO Scientific
Hatboro, Pa.

ROCHE MEDICAL ELECTRONICS, INC
Cranbury, N.J.

Morris Rossman, DO,
Chairman, Department of Cardiology
Delaware Valley Medical Center
Bristol, Pa.

Nanette K. Wenger, MD,
Professor of Medicine (Cardiology)
Emory University School of Medicine
Director, Cardiac Clinics
Grady Memorial Hospital
Atlanta, Ga.

Also the staffs of:

ALBERT EINSTEIN MEDICAL CENTER
Daroff Division
Philadelphia, Pa.

ALBERT EINSTEIN MEDICAL CENTER
Northern Division
Philadelphia, Pa.

DELAWARE VALLEY MEDICAL CENTER
Bristol, Pa.

HAHNEMANN MEDICAL COLLEGE & HOSPITAL
Philadelphia, Pa.

HOSPITAL OF THE UNIVERSITY OF PENNSYLVANIA
Department of Radiology
Philadelphia, Pa.
Ronald Arenson, MD

How serum enzyme levels change after myocardial infarction

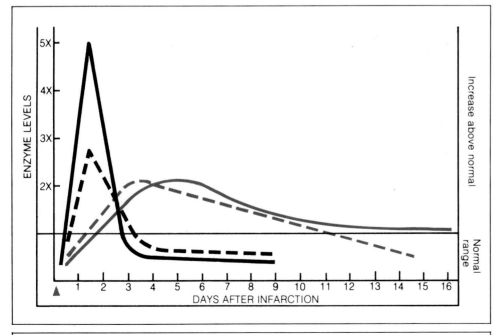

| HBD —— | SGOT ▬ ▬ ▬ | CPK ▬▬ | LDH – – – | Onset of chest pain ▲ |

Selected references

Books

Abels, Linda F. MOSBY'S MANUAL OF CRITICAL CARE: PRACTICES AND PROCEDURES, NINETEEN SEVENTY-NINE. St. Louis: C.V. Mosby Co., 1979.

Andreoli, Kathleen, et al. COMPREHENSIVE CARDIAC CARE: A TEXT FOR NURSES AND OTHER HEALTH PRACTITIONERS, 4th ed. St. Louis: C.V. Mosby Co., 1979.

Bolooki, Hooshang. CLINICAL APPLICATION OF INTRA-AORTIC BALLOON PUMP. Mount Kisco, N.Y.: Futura Publishing Co., 1977.

Braunwald, Eugene. HEART DISEASE: A TEXTBOOK OF CARDIOVASCULAR MEDICINE, 2 vols. Philadelphia: W.B. Saunders Co., 1980.

Brunner, Lillian S. THE LIPPINCOTT MANUAL OF NURSING PRACTICE, 2nd ed. Philadelphia: J.B. Lippincott Co., 1978.

Brunner, Lillian S., et al. TEXTBOOK OF MEDICAL-SURGICAL NURSING, 4th ed. Philadelphia: J.B. Lippincott Co., 1980.

Burrell, Zeb, Jr., and Lennette O. Burrell. CRITICAL CARE, 3rd ed. St. Louis: C.V. Mosby Co., 1977.

Comoss, Patricia M., et al. CARDIAC REHABILITATION: A COMPREHENSIVE NURSING APPROACH. Philadelphia: J.B. Lippincott Co., 1979.

DEALING WITH EMERGENCIES. NURSING PHOTOBOOK™ Series. Springhouse, Pa.: Intermed Communications, Inc., 1980.

Disch, Joann M. DIAGNOSTIC PROCEDURES FOR CARDIOVASCULAR DISEASE. New York: Appleton-Century-Crofts, 1979.

Fink, Burton W. CONGENITAL HEART DISEASE: A DEDUCTIVE APPROACH TO ITS DIAGNOSIS. Chicago: Year Book Medical Publishers, Inc. 1975.

Hurst, J. Willis, and R. Bruce Logue, eds. THE HEART, 3rd ed. New York: McGraw-Hill Book Co.,1974.

Jones, Patricia. CARDIAC PACING. New York: Appleton-Century-Crofts, 1980.

Meltzer, L.E., et al. INTENSIVE CORONARY CARE: A MANUAL FOR NURSES, 3rd ed. Bowie, Md.: Charles Press Publishers, 1977.

Moss, Arthur J., et al. HEART DISEASE IN INFANTS AND ADOLESCENTS, 2nd ed. Baltimore: Williams & Wilkins Co., 1977.

Naughton, John, and Herman K. Hellerstein, eds. EXERCISE TESTING AND EXERCISE TRAINING IN CORONARY HEART DISEASE. New York: Academic Press, 1973.

NURSING DRUG HANDBOOK™. *Nursing82* Books. Springhouse, Pa.: Intermed Communications, Inc.,1981.

Perloff, Joseph K. THE CLINICAL RECOGNITION OF CONGENITAL HEART DISEASE, 2nd ed. Philadelphia: W.B. Saunders Co., 1978.

PROVIDING RESPIRATORY CARE. NURSING PHOTOBOOK™ Series. Springhouse, Pa.: Intermed Communications, Inc., 1979.

Redman, Barbara K. THE PROCESS OF PATIENT TEACHING IN NURSING, 3rd ed. St. Louis: C.V. Mosby Co.,1978.

Sade, Robert M. INFANT AND CHILD CARE IN HEART SURGERY. Chicago: Year Book Medical Publishers, Inc., 1977.

Storlie, Frances. PATIENT TEACHING IN CRITICAL CARE. New York: Appleton-Century-Crofts, 1970.

USING MONITORS. NURSING PHOTOBOOK™ Series. Springhouse, Pa.: Intermed Communications, Inc., 1980.

Vince, Dennis J. ESSENTIALS OF PEDIATRIC CARDIOLOGY. Philadelphia: J.B. Lippincott, Co., 1973.

Wenger, Nanette K., and Herman K. Hellerstein. REHABILITATION OF THE CORONARY PATIENT. New York: John Wiley & Sons, 1978.

Wilson, Philip K., et al. POLICIES AND PROCEDURES OF A CARDIAC REHABILITATION PROGRAM: IMMEDIATE TO LONG-TERM CARE. Philadelphia: Lea & Febiger, 1978.

Periodicals

Bricker, Patricia Lee. *The Intensive Nursing Demands of the Intra-aortic Balloon Pump,* RN. 43:22-29, July 1980.

Furman, Seymour. *Recent Developments in Cardiac Pacing,* HEART & LUNG. 7:813-826, September/October 1978.

Hammond, Cecile E. *Protecting Patients with Temporary Transvenous Pacemakers,* NURSING78. 8:82-86, November 1978.

Manwaring, Mary. *What Patients Need to Know about Pacemakers,* AMERICAN JOURNAL OF NURSING. 77:825-830, May 1977.

Rossel, Carol L., and I.B. Alyn. *Living with a Permanent Pacemaker,* HEART & LUNG. 6:273-279, March/April 1977.

Sweetwood, Hannelore. *Patients with Pacemakers,* NURSING77. 7:44-51, March 1977.

Théroux, P., et al. *Prognostic Value of Exercise Testing Soon After Myocardial Infarction,* NEW ENGLAND JOURNAL OF MEDICINE. 301:341-345, August 16, 1979.

Watts, R.J. *Symposium on Teaching and Rehabilitating the Cardiac Patient,* NURSING CLINICS OF NORTH AMERICA. 11:349-359, June 1976.

Whitman, Gayle. *Intra-aortic Balloon Pumping and Cardiac Mechanics: A Programmed Lesson,* HEART & LUNG. 7:1034-1050, November/December 1978.

Winslow, E.H., and T.M. Weber. *Rehabilitation of the Cardiac Patient. Progressive Exercise to Combat the Hazards of Bed Rest,* AMERICAN JOURNAL OF NURSING. 80:349-359, June 1976.

Selected references for the patient with a heart condition

Burrows, Susan G., and Carole A. Gassert. MOVING RIGHT ALONG...AFTER OPEN HEART SURGERY. Atlanta: Pritchett & Hull Associates, Inc., 1979.

Cambre, Suzanne. THE SENSUOUS HEART: GUIDELINES FOR SEX AFTER A HEART ATTACK. Atlanta: Pritchett & Hull Associates, Inc., 1978.

Cohn, Keith, et al. COMING BACK: A GUIDE TO RECOVERING FROM HEART ATTACK AND LIVING CONFIDENTLY WITH CORONARY DISEASE. Reading, Mass.: Addison-Wesley Publishing Co., 1979.

Purcell, Julia Ann, et al. ANGINA PECTORIS. Atlanta: Pritchett & Hull Associates, Inc., 1979.

Purcell, Julia Ann, and Barbara Johnston. A STRONGER PUMP. Atlanta: Pritchett & Hull Associates, Inc., 1980.

Snider, Arthur J. A DOCTOR DISCUSSES LEARNING HOW TO LIVE WITH HEART TROUBLE. Chicago: Budlong Press Co., 1976.

Available from the American Heart Association, 7320 Greenville Ave., Dallas, TX 75231:
    AN OLDER PERSON'S GUIDE TO CARDIOVASCULAR HEALTH
    HEART ATTACK: HOW TO REDUCE YOUR RISK
    THE HEART AND BLOOD VESSELS
    IF YOUR CHILD HAS A CONGENITAL HEART DEFECT
    LIVING WITH ANGINA
    LIVING WITH YOUR PACEMAKER
    RECIPES FOR FAT-CONTROLLED, LOW-CHOLESTEROL MEALS

Available from the Department of Health, Education, and Welfare, Washington, DC 20203:
    CALLING IT QUITS. Publication No. 79-1824
    MEDICINE FOR THE LAYMAN: HEART ATTACKS. Publication No. 80-1803
    WHY DO YOU SMOKE? Publication No. 79-1822

Index

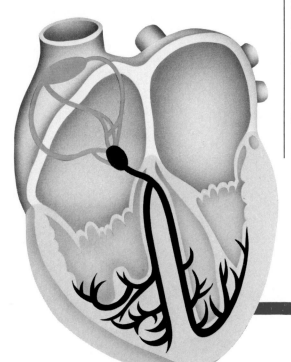

Index

T

U

V

W

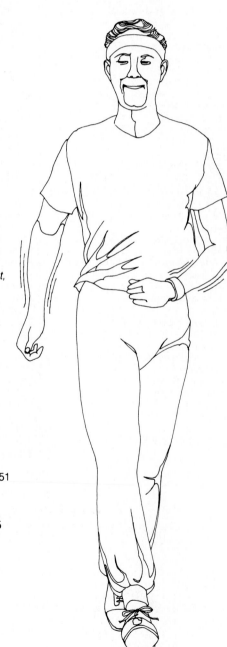